HIDDEN Food Allergies

> ❝Finding out what I'm allergic to with t...
> transformed my life. For the first time in thirt...
> —Denise Lewis, Olympic gold medal winner and star of the hit B... ...uy Come Dancing

❝I feel so much better. I'm nowhere as tired. I have no bloating.
My eczema is a lot better. And I've even lost a couple of pounds.❞
—Liza

❝I've definitely lost weight and am much less bloated. People have noticed
I've got my waist back and I'm in trousers I haven't worn for years.
My constipation has completely gone. I used to use my inhaler four times
a day, now I don't use it at all. Overall I feel so much better.❞
—Katie

❝My energy is better and I'm more alert. My irritable bowel has been
better and I have a lot less trapped gas. I used to get tired after a meal—
and I would get the feeling of still being hungry. I don't get that so
much anymore. I would often get more pain after eating.
That's reduced, too. Overall I feel really good.❞
—Leanne

❝I can't tell you how much better I feel. I'm 100 percent. Having
the food intolerance blood test has been the best thing I've done.
It has transformed my health. I have lost the entire 140 pounds that
I'd put on over the past three years. I wish I'd done it sooner!❞
—Rebecca

❝Within a week of cutting all dairy products from his diet,
my hyperactive seven-year-old was less excitable, more settled,
and could concentrate better so he is now doing much better in school.
His chronic insomnia has gone and he now sleeps through the night.
He doesn't need the steroid medication for his asthma anymore.❞
—Iain's mom

❝Within a week I was going to the bathroom every two days
(instead of weekly), my bloated stomach was gone, and I was down to a
size 10 from a size 14. My lethargy was caused by the yeasty foods I ate.
I've gone from 156 to 129 pounds, and look so much trimmer now.❞
—Joanne

"Within a couple of days of cutting these foods out of my diet, I began to feel better. My head felt clearer, my energy levels and sinusitis improved, and even my rheumatoid arthritis pain eased considerably. After ten years of frequent and severe headaches and migraines, I am pleased to say that these have also dramatically reduced."

—*Alison*

"Life is now free of pain and medication and I have complete mobility. I am amazed at the difference in my quality of life simply by making such simple adjustments."

—*John*

"About ten days after starting the diet I noticed I was less tired in the morning. Now I'm not tired at all when I wake up. I have loads more energy, I'm less bored, I'm concentrating better and I feel a lot happier. I'm getting on better at school and concentrating better in class. I'm also doing more activities and sports, I'm a lot calmer than I used to be and I'm not getting into trouble at school anymore. I feel more positive about my future. I'm going to stay on the diet for life. It's brilliant!"

—*Liam*

"I started feeling better after one week on the diet. For three years I had suffered with joint pain and swelling in my hands, ankles, and arms, shooting pains in my arms and legs, fluid retention, extreme fatigue, uncontrollable food cravings, heartburn, chronic skin rashes, and heart palpitations despite taking several prescription medications. By seven weeks later all of my symptoms had gone and I had stopped all my medication. I also lost 15 pounds."

—*Cathy*

"My lifelong lethargy has lifted, I've lost all my constipation, bloatedness, and pain. I am simply delighted."

—*Sandra*

"This book beautifully explains how food allergy and intolerance is responsible for much widespread chronic poor health today. As well as being an invaluable tool for those wanting to manage their condition, this is required reading for every clinician."

—*Maureen Jenkins, Trustee of Allergy UK and from Sussex Allergy Advice*

HIDDEN
Food Allergies

HIDDEN
Food Allergies

The Essential Guide to
Uncovering Hidden Food Allergies—
and Achieving Permanent Relief

JAMES BRALY, M.D.,
& PATRICK HOLFORD

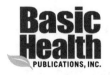

**Basic
Health**
PUBLICATIONS, INC.

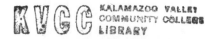

The information contained in this book is based upon the research and personal and professional experiences of the authors. It is not intended as a substitute for consulting with your physician or other healthcare provider. Any attempt to diagnose and treat an illness should be done under the direction of a healthcare professional.

The publisher does not advocate the use of any particular healthcare protocol but believes the information in this book should be available to the public. The publisher and authors are not responsible for any adverse effects or consequences resulting from the use of the suggestions, preparations, or procedures discussed in this book. Should the reader have any questions concerning the appropriateness of any procedures or preparation mentioned, the authors and the publisher strongly suggest consulting a professional healthcare advisor.

Basic Health Publications, Inc.
28812 Top of the World Drive
Laguna Beach, CA 92651
949-715-7327 • www.basichealthpub.com

First published in Great Britain in December 2005 by
Piatkus Books Ltd., 5 Windmill Street, London W1T 2JA

Library of Congress Cataloging-in-Publication Data

Braly, James.
    Hidden food allergies : the essential guide to uncovering hidden food
allergies—and achieving permanent relief / James Braly and Patrick Holford.
        p. cm.
    Rev. ed. of: Hidden food allergies / Patrick Holford and James Braley. 2005.
    Includes bibliographical references and index.
    ISBN-13: 978-1-59120-195-3
    ISBN-10: 1-59120-195-0
    1. Food allergy—Popular works. I. Holford, Patrick. II. Holford, Patrick.
Hidden food allergies. III. Title.

    RC596.B728   2006
    616.97'5—dc22

                                                    2006019737

In-house Editor: Tara Durkin
Typesetting and Book design: Gary A. Rosenberg
Cover Design: Mike Stromberg

Printed in the United States of America

10   9   8   7   6   5   4   3   2   1

Contents

Introduction

————◄○►————

Finding and Losing Your Hidden Food Allergies

How are you feeling, right at this moment? The odds are that it's well below your potential for pain-free, symptom-free, high-energy living—and all for a simple reason. You are eating or drinking something that doesn't suit you and that your immune system is trying to reject.

Your reaction to what you eat may not be immediate or severe. But it could be insidiously adding to your burden of unwellness, with the potential to tip over into chronic, serious health problems such as irritable bowel syndrome, migraine, depression, chronic fatigue, addictive overeating, or asthma.

Of course, there are other allergens—airborne substances such as pollen, or dust mites or cat dander (flakes of the animals' skin). Chemicals in food, household products, or the environment can be culprits, too. The most common, however, is food.

Officially, an estimated one in three of us have an allergy, according to a survey by the Royal College of Physicians.[1] But this could be a serious underestimate. In Europe, allergy is considered to be the number one chronic illness. According to Warren Filley, M.D., of the American College of Allergy, Asthma, and Immunology, "38 percent of Americans suffer from allergies, twice as many as experts previously thought" (November 1999). And in one survey of 3,300 adults, 43 percent said that they experienced adverse reactions to food.[2] In another, 70 percent of people suffering from a wide range of chronic illnesses discussed in this book, who had failed to respond to conventional treatment, found relief from their symptoms by identifying their food allergies and avoiding those foods.[3] Almost a quarter obtained 100 percent relief!

In our experience, the vast majority of people—and unfortunately most of their family physicians—have no idea their health problems may be related to eating specific foods. Most people's food allergies are truly hidden from them.

The truth is that the majority of people, including you, are likely to suffer

1

for years not only not knowing they have an allergy—but also, not knowing how to treat it by identifying which foods they react to and how to regain their tolerance to those foods. Our personal stories are a case in point.

WE'VE BEEN THERE . . .

I (James Braly) suffered from severe, disabling migraines as a child—so severe that my left eye crossed and the pupil dilated. It was only as an adult that I finally discovered I was allergic to dairy products. Gluten grains—wheat, rye, and barley products in particular—were also causing nasal congestion, skin rashes when I ran long distances, extreme bloating, and sleepiness after eating, and on rare occasions muscle spasms in my air passages, causing them to temporarily close shut and my breathing to become extremely difficult. Ironically, wheat and cow's milk were my favorite food groups throughout my childhood and adolescence. I went for many years without suspecting either to be the underlying cause of my symptoms. Now, with much less dairy and no gluten grains in my diet, I remain free of migraines, nasal congestion, hives, and chronic breathing problems.

I (Patrick Holford) also suffered throughout my childhood and adolescence from migraines, sinus problems, and ear infections. I saw countless doctors and specialists, had my adenoids and tonsils removed, and had two sinus operations, numerous courses of antibiotics, and many nights of excruciating pain from migraines—only to discover that I was allergic to milk and yeast.

Your symptoms may be more or less severe than ours, and caused by factors other than food allergies. Chances are, however, that food intolerances or allergies are adding to your burden, and in many cases, are proving to be the main cause of any health problems. This constitutes unnecessary suffering, and as we don't want you to have to struggle with it any longer, we have written this book to guide you through the maze of discovering which foods make you ill and what to eat instead. We'll let you know about the amazing scientific advances that mean you can now identify food allergies with simple blood tests, including a pinprick of blood using a simple home test kit.

What's more, we'll explain why you become sensitive or intolerant to certain foods by revealing the underlying causes of most food allergies, and how to eliminate these causes and thereby reduce your allergic potential. We'll explain how to "desensitize" yourself to most of the foods you're allergic to so you can eat them once more, a process that usually takes just three months.

Some types of food allergies, of course, are for life—peanut, shellfish, and wheat (gluten) allergies come to mind here. If you have this kind, you can't desensitize yourself completely. They are often genetically linked, fixed, and permanent food allergies, remaining potential dangers for a lifetime and need to be avoided.

HOW TO USE THIS BOOK

But first, here's an overview of what you'll find in this book. Chapter 1 helps you discover if your health problems are likely to be caused or aggravated by something you are eating and, if so, whether that is triggering a food allergy, food sensitivity, or food intolerance. Chapter 2 explains the two main types of food allergy: immediate-onset "IgE based" allergy, and the much more prevalent delayed or hidden "IgG-based" food allergy. Chapter 3 runs through the most common health problems associated with food allergy.

If you've got children, Chapter 4 lets you know how to prevent and solve childhood allergies, and the common health problems they cause. Chapter 5 presents new, exciting findings, namely the relationship between food allergies, food addiction, and alcoholism. Chapter 6 goes through the top twenty common food allergens. Chapter 7 tells you how to identify which foods you arc allergic to, while Chapter 8 explains the basis for correcting the underlying causes that lead to allergy in the first place. Finally, Chapter 9 gives you a clear action plan for relief from food allergies, then segues into the appendices. Here, you'll find useful information on food families (so if you're allergic to one food, you can make informed choices about eating any of its "relatives"), a symptom score chart, an "Abstinence Symptom Severity Scale" (frequently used by Dr. Braly to monitor response to addiction therapy and risk of relapse), and detailed information on the severe gluten allergy, celiac disease.

Throughout, our promise to you is this: we will help you improve your health by finding out which foods suit you and which foods trigger an allergic reaction, show you how to desensitize yourself to most all of those foods, and give you the know-how to achieve *permanent* allergy relief. And all without the need for prescription and over-the-counter medication or unnecessarily restrictive diets.

Wishing you the best of allergy-free health!

Chapter 1

——◁○▷——

Is What You Eat Making You Ill?

If you have nagging or serious health problems that come and go, or are worse after eating certain foods, better on holiday or vacations when your diet is different, or unresponsive to conventional medical treatment, now is a good moment to question whether something you are eating is making you ill.

Most major health problems—diabetes, heart disease, even Alzheimer's disease and most types of cancer—are now recognized as primarily diet related. So why shouldn't headaches, depression, anxiety, asthma, digestive problems, joint aches, fatigue, or whatever it is you are suffering from be diet related?

In most cases, they are. There may, of course, be other contributory factors; but finding out which foods suit you and which foods don't can make a massive difference to how you feel.

THREE TYPICAL STORIES

To show how this works, we asked Britain's most watched breakfast television franchise, GMTV—for which coauthor Patrick Holford is nutrition expert—to give us three volunteers with different health problems who had had no relief from conventional, drug-oriented medicine, and to allow us three weeks to find out whether food was making them ill.

Liza, the first, had suffered from eczema since early childhood. She also felt tired a lot of the time, and suffered from occasional bloating and weight fluctuations. She kept her eczema under control with a cortisone-based cream, but her hands were still crinkly and sore. She also drank coffee or caffeinated drinks throughout the day to keep her awake.

The second, Katie, had all the classic symptoms of irritable bowel syndrome—bloating, abdominal pain, constipation, and occasional diarrhea. She also had asthma and used an inhaler several times each day. She had gained 28

5

pounds in weight and gone up two dress sizes. Her doctor had given her a type of fiber to help with her constipation, but it didn't help. She suspected that she was reacting to certain foods but didn't know what.

The third was Leanne. Chronically tired, Leanne thought wheat made her worse and had avoided it. But she still felt exhausted most of the time, and on top of that had migraines, a poor sex drive, and digestive problems. She'd been tested for thyroid problems and glandular fever, but she was told that there was no conventional medical diagnosis or treatment for her condition.

We tested each volunteer for food allergy with a simple home test kit using a pinprick of blood. Liza, we found, was strongly allergic to dairy products; Katie was allergic to yeast, almonds, and cashews; and Leanne had multiple food allergies. As well as giving general advice about healthy eating, they were each given some specific supplements such as multivitamins, digestive enzymes, probiotics (friendly bacteria), and the amino acid glutamine. Due to caffeine's role in contributing to poor sleep and chronic fatigue, Liza was advised to quit all caffeine.

Here's what happened, in their own words, three weeks later.

Liza: I feel so much better. Nothing like as tired. I am really surprised at how easy I found it to cut out the caffeine, and I have more energy, not less. The milk avoidance itself wasn't so difficult, but I was amazed to find out how many foods had hidden milk; so it took a week to discover what I could and couldn't have. Overall, it's been fine. I have no bloating. My skin is a lot better. I have no sores or cuts. I have lost a couple of pounds.

Katie: People have noticed I've got my waist back. I'm in trousers I haven't worn for years. I am much less bloated. I've had very few stomach cramps. I've definitely lost weight. I went out for dinner at an Indian restaurant and had no reaction. I'm also using my inhaler much less. I used to use my inhaler four times a day, now none. One day I inadvertently had some muesli with almonds, one of my allergy foods. I felt itchy after that. My constipation has completely gone. Used to go once a week and suffer stomach pains in between. Now I go every day. Overall, I feel so much better.

Leanne: My energy is better and I'm more alert. My irritable bowel has been OK, better, not dramatic, although I do have a lot less gas pain. I don't get so tired. I used to get tired after a meal—I would get the feeling of still being hungry. I don't get that so much any more. I would often get more pain after eating. That's reduced, too. Overall, I feel really good but there's still room for improvement.

These three cases show how important it is to pinpoint precisely what foods you're allergic to. Simply put, a food allergy means your immune system is producing antibodies designed to attack certain proteins you eat, causing symptoms. And that's what was happening to Liza when she consumed dairy products.

WHEN IT'S NOT AN ALLERGY . . .

We'll be exploring allergies in depth in the next chapter, but first let's take a look at the other ways food can affect your well-being.

Food Intolerance Is Not a Food Allergy

As we've seen, Liza coped with exhaustion by guzzling coffee and caffeinated drinks. Little did she know that the caffeine was actually making her more tired. Some foods or drinks knock your system out of balance, often interfering with sound, restful sleep, and two of the big culprits are sugar and caffeine (also present in tea and soft drinks). The more of these you eat or drink, the more resistant you may become to their effects, resulting in rebound exhaustion. This is an intolerance, not an allergy.

There are other kinds of food intolerance that we define as a non-immunological response to a food—that is, you get symptoms, but there's no observable or measurable immune reaction. The most common example is intolerance of lactose—milk sugar, found in cow's milk—which happens in people who lack adequate supplies of the enzyme lactase, which is needed to digest it. This kind of intolerance means milk is hard to digest—a very different thing from an allergy to cow's milk, where the immune reaction can cause inflammation (in Liza's case, resulting in eczema). Lactose intolerance and milk allergy do often go hand in hand, however.

Food/Chemical Sensitivity Is Not a Food Allergy

Some people—often those who also have food allergies—are especially sensitive to certain chemicals added to food. Their symptoms can be very similar to allergic reactions, and often may include hives or urticaria, which are mosquito-bite-like, itchy eruptions on the skin. In children with chronic hives, sensitivity to a food additive such as food colorings, preservatives, emulsifiers, or taste enhancers is often a cause. A recent double-blind, placebo-controlled study showed that three out of every four children with chronic hives greatly improved within two weeks on a food-additive-free diet, while half the children had complete relief by six months.[1] If, however, you or your child suffers from hives that don't improve on avoiding additives, we recommend that you investigate food allergies as a probable cause.

Five common additives that often provoke symptoms are:

- **MSG (monosodium glutamate)** is a taste enhancer found in Chinese food, much of restaurant fast food, and many tinned or packaged foods. Symptoms can include nausea, vomiting, headaches, and dizziness. Glutamate is a natural brain chemical that, when excessive, is toxic to brain nerve cells.

- **Sulfites/metasulfites/metabisulfites** are used to maintain freshness, are common in factory-prepared foods and white wines, and often added to potatoes, avocados, shellfish, greens, and vegetables in restaurant salad bars. Asthmatics may have severe reactions to sulfites. Sulfite sensitivity may be associated with a molybdenum trace mineral deficiency.

- **Tartrazine** (FD&C Yellow No. 5) is used widely as a food coloring and is known to cause hyperactivity, migraines, and asthmatic attacks. It also depletes the body of vitamin B_6 and zinc.

- **BHA** is used as a preservative, especially in foods containing fats such as deli and lunch meats. It can cause hives and other skin reactions.

- **Inulin**, extracted from artichokes, and its chemical cousin oligofructose are now added to an increasing number of industrially processed foods, such as sweets, drinks, yogurt, ice cream, chocolate, butter, and breakfast cereals. It can cause allergy-like symptoms, such as breathing difficulties, in susceptible people.

While we won't be covering chemical sensitivity any further than this, we do not mean to communicate that they are not important causes of human suffering. They are. We strongly recommend that everyone avoids food containing these additives as much as possible.

Food Poisoning Is Not a Food Allergy

Food poisoning—most commonly characterized by nausea, vomiting, and diarrhea—is a widespread and serious problem with a number of causes. (In rare cases, food poisoning can lead to death.) Some plants and animals are simply unsafe for human consumption. For example, the "death cap" family of mushrooms can trigger severe or even fatal poisoning. A more common source is spoiled or improperly cooked food. Chicken, for instance, can be rife with "bad" bacteria such as salmonella, and uncooked fish can be contaminated with bacteria such as *Listeria* or *Clostridium botulinum,* which causes botulism.

There are about 76 million cases of food poisoning annually in the United States, and food poisoning is associated with 5,000 deaths. In Britain alone there are 100,000 reported cases of food poisoning a year, but probably over twenty times that number go unreported, often because the symptoms don't always develop immediately and affected people fail to realize it's caused by something they ate, or don't go to the doctor. People often assume they are allergic to shellfish, for example, when they may have no allergy but have had a bout of food poisoning.

Nutritional Deficiency Is Not a Food Allergy

Another possible reason why what you're eating is making you ill is simply that it's poor-quality food, lacking in nutrients. Say you live on processed food, or convenient, fast ("trash") foods, and don't consume much fruit, vegetables, or whole foods (that is, beans, lentils, nuts, seeds, brown rice, or whole-grain breads and pastas). If that's you, you may find yourself feeling tired, "toxic," and unwell because you're simply not getting the vitamins, minerals, and other key nutrients your mind and body need.

We recommend a widely varied, well-balanced, nutrient-dense diet, with an abundance of (nonallergic) fruits and vegetables, nuts, seeds, legumes, fish, and meats, and a basic daily oral supplement program for everybody to ensure optimum nutrition, and to make you less prone to developing an allergy (see Chapter 9).

ARE YOU SUFFERING FROM A HIDDEN FOOD ALLERGY?

We've now looked at a number of food-related reactions. But what if your problems with a food or foods don't match up? Let's examine the classic symptoms of a food allergy now, to discover whether this is what you're suffering from.

The symptoms below are the most common signs of increased likelihood for food allergy. Score 1 point for each "yes" answer.

YOUR INSTANT ALLERGY CHECK

☐ Are you chronically tired?

☐ Can you gain weight in hours?

☐ Do you get bloated after eating, having to loosen your belt a notch or two?

☐ Do you suffer from diarrhea or constipation?

☐ Do you suffer from abdominal pain?

THE TELLTALE SIGNS OF FOOD ALLERGY

One of the telltale signs that you might be allergic to something you're eating is that the symptoms come and go. One day you feel fine; the next your joints are aching, or you've got a headache, are blocked up or bloated, and you don't know why. Since most food allergies are delayed (we will discuss this in Chapter 2), symptoms often only develop hours or even days after eating the food, making it difficult to put two and two together. (Even more confusing, eating the food you're allergic to can make you temporarily feel better, and only later become problematic. We will discuss this further in Chapter 5.)

Another sign is that you feel better when your diet changes dramatically. For example, if you go on an exotic holiday and eat foods you never usually do, you may, by chance, exclude a food to which you are allergic. (Of course, there are other reasons why you might feel better on holiday: you might be less stressed, for instance.)

Yet most people never vary their menus, and eat the same favorite foods every single day. In our clinics we have seen hundreds of patients whose whole lives have been allergic reactions. For as long as they can remember, they've felt tired or bloated, and suffered from depression, fatigue, headaches, asthma, eczema, or other classic allergic symptoms. And every day of their lives, like most Americans, they've eaten wheat or dairy products—classic, extremely common allergens.

It's impossible to know how well you can feel if you've never felt that good. Cathy B. is a case in point. For three years Cathy suffered from joint pain and swelling in her hands, ankles, and arms, shooting pains in her arms and legs, unexplained weight gain and fluid retention, extreme fatigue (despite sleeping up to sixteen hours a day), uncontrollable food cravings, heartburn, skin rash, and heart palpitations despite taking several prescription medications. An IgG food allergy test (see page 74) showed that she was reacting to several foods, specifically dairy, eggs, sugar cane, yeast, bananas, and scallops. She immediately cut all of these foods out of her diet. During the first days off these foods she had a terrible "killer headache" (that is, a withdrawal headache). Gradually her symptoms began to abate. Within one week she definitely felt better and after seven weeks of following the diet, Cathy was symptom- and medication-free. She had also lost 15 pounds without counting calories. Once during this time, she broke the diet and the next day many of her symptoms returned, fortunately only temporarily.

☐ Do you sometimes get really sleepy right after eating?

☐ Do you suffer from nasal congestion, sneezing, running nose, and so on?

☐ Do you suffer from rashes, itches, asthma, or shortness of breath?

☐ Do you have recurrent colds, sore throats, or sinus problems?

☐ Do you suffer from water retention, with swelling under your eyes, or swollen fingers or ankles?

☐ Do you suffer from headaches or migraines?

☐ Do you suffer from occasional muscle or joint aches or pains, possibly after eating certain foods?

☐ Do you suffer from "brain fog" or patches of inexplicable depression?

☐ Do you get better on holidays abroad, when your diet is completely different?

Any "yes" answer to these questions means there's a real possibility that you have an allergy. If you score four or more "yes's," it's pretty much guaranteed.

Now, let's take a closer look at the two main kinds of food allergies.

Chapter 2

-----◄○►-----

Immediate- and Delayed-Onset Food Allergies

If you were to unfold and lay your small intestine flat on the ground, its inside surface area would equal that of a tennis court! This selective barrier is the gateway between your body and the outside world—it is your "inner skin." Only food substances such as vitamins, minerals, amino acids from digested proteins, and so on are allowed through—at least in theory. The police force guarding your inner gateway is your immune system.

FOOD AS INVADER

A food allergy develops when your immune system treats a food you've eaten as an invader, not a friend. This can happen for a number of reasons. In some cases, the food may contain a kind of protein that the body doesn't like. For example, many people's immune system will react to gliadin, a protein abundant in wheat, rye, and barley. This is most often an inherited condition (about 1 percent of the American adult population—3 million people—are sensitive to gliadin and don't know it).

In most cases, food allergies develop when the inside lining of the digestive tract becomes permeable or abnormally "leaky" because of antibiotic use, excess alcohol consumption, use of aspirin substitutes like Aleve or ibuprofen, gut infection, excessive physical or emotional stress, or other reasons. (We'll discuss these more in Chapter 8 when we show you how to decrease your allergic potential.) The leakiness enables incompletely digested food proteins to "gatecrash" your bloodstream, and your immune system will react to these outright strangers by attacking them.

This reaction happens on a number of fronts. Your immune system attaches the equivalent of handcuffs, called antibodies, to the invading foods. The immune system then attacks and digests them with specialized cells such as phagocytes; and releases all sorts of reactive chemicals, such as histamine, which also cause many of the sudden and chronic symptoms we experience as allergic reactions.

The two most common types of allergic reaction to foods, namely the immediate-onset and the much more common delayed-onset, involve two different families of antibodies, called IgE and IgG respectively. The "Ig" stands for immunoglobulin, while "E" or "G" is the type or family of immunoglobulin. Let's take a closer look at these two different kinds of allergies to see whether or not you are likely to have one.

IMMEDIATE-ONSET FOOD ALLERGIES (IgE)

The best-known and most studied form of food allergy involves the IgE family of antibodies, and is also known as a type 1, immediate-onset, or atopic food allergy. These allergies are considered "classic" partly because they were documented in medicine first, and partly because of the immediate and obvious reaction they involve. These are the allergies you read about in the newspaper, when someone dies from eating shellfish or peanuts.

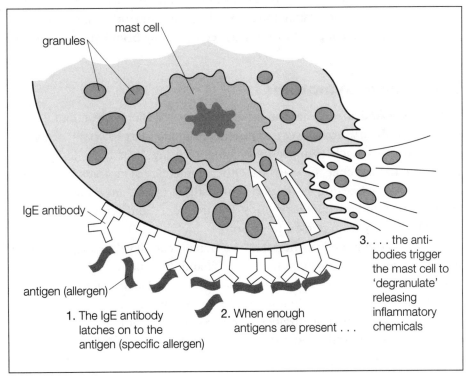

Figure 2.1. How IgE food allergies happen.

However, immediate-onset allergies are relatively rare: fewer than 5 percent of us have them, and they are found mostly in children. If you are one of the 2 in 100 adults to have an IgE allergy, you almost certainly know about it because the reactions usually involve only one or two foods and appear within seconds or up to only two hours later. So the condition is usually self-diagnosed and you will already have stopped eating the foods in question.

Immediate-onset allergies can be genetic: you can inherit a tendency to manufacture a specific type of IgE antibody to certain foods. This is why a very serious and common gluten allergy, celiac disease, runs in families (we discuss celiac disease in more detail in later chapters, and in Appendix 4).

Here's how IgE food allergies happen. One side of the IgE antibody is designed to recognize and tenaciously bind to the food allergen. Before this happens, however, the other side of the IgE antibody must become attached to a troublesome, unstable immune cell called a mast cell. Mast cells are found almost everywhere in the human body, but are especially concentrated in the lining of your digestive tract. Primed for action, the IgE-coated mast cells patiently wait for the food allergen to appear.

When you eat that food, the IgE antibodies on the surface of mast cells hungrily latch onto it. Instantaneously, histamine and other allergy-related chemicals come gushing out of the mast cells, rapidly bringing on a range of nasty symptoms.

The Classic Symptoms

The skin, gut, and airways are the usual arena for IgE allergic reactions. So you may see a rash, urticaria (hives), or eczema. You may start to vomit, or experience nausea, stomach cramps, dull aching, bloating, heartburn, indigestion, constipation, flatulence, or diarrhea. Other immediate symptoms include the coughing and wheezing associated with asthma or the sneezing and stuffy nose of a person with allergic rhinitis. The frequency and severity of the reactions vary greatly from person to person.

At the extreme end of the scale, the person can develop anaphylaxis—a reaction where the throat and mouth swell and difficulty breathing suddenly appears, resulting in death from suffocation. Anaphylactic reactions can also include redness of the skin, itching or hives, rapid dropping of blood pressure, an irregular, fast heartbeat, dizziness, faintness, and loss of consciousness.

Here are some of the more common conditions in which IgE food allergy may play a part:

• Allergic dermatitis, eczema

- Angioedema (deep swelling of the skin, for example, on the mouth, face, lips, and throat)
- Anaphylaxis (severe and dangerous allergic reaction)
- Asthma
- Hay fever (seasonal allergic rhinitis)
- Hives (urticaria)

On top of identifying and avoiding allergens, there are other ways of reducing your allergic potential, and the amount of histamine released, without resorting to anti-allergic medication. We'll discuss these in Chapter 8.

DELAYED-ONSET FOOD ALLERGY (IgG)

IgG allergic reactions are much more common than the IgE type in both children and adults, affecting as many as one in three people—and particularly among those with chronic conditions unresponsive to conventional medicine, up to 70 percent or more.

These food allergies occur when your immune system creates an overabundance of IgG antibodies to a particular food allergen. The antibodies, instead of attaching to mast cells like their IgE counterparts, bind directly to the food particles as they enter your bloodstream, creating "immune complex-

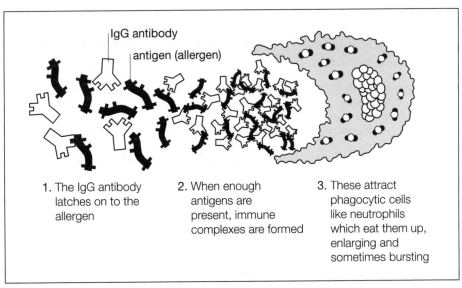

1. The IgG antibody latches on to the allergen

2. When enough antigens are present, immune complexes are formed

3. These attract phagocytic cells like neutrophils which eat them up, enlarging and sometimes bursting

Figure 2.2. How IgG food allergies happen.

es." The more of these you have floating around the bloodstream, the more on edge your immune system becomes, sending out phagocytes to gobble the complexes up. Basically, your immune system gradually goes into red alert.

This process takes time, which is why IgG symptoms are delayed and only appear two hours to several days after consuming the food allergen. For example, a migraine headache characteristically appears forty-eight hours after the allergen is eaten.

Unlike immediate food reactions, these delayed reactions can involve almost any organ or tissue in the human body, potentially provoking over 100 allergic symptoms, and are implicated in well over 100 medical diseases and conditions. Here is a partial list of the more common conditions caused or aggravated by IgG food allergy. (We'll be discussing many of these conditions in more detail in the next chapter.)

- Allergic rhinitis, nonseasonal

- Ankylosing spondylitis (disabling arthritis of the spine)

- Anxiety, panic attacks (involves food allergen changes in brain chemistry)

- Asthma (may involve both IgG and IgE antibodies at the same time)

- Attention deficit hyperactivity disorder (ADHD) (involves food allergen changes in brain chemistry)

- Autism (commonly associated with milk and gluten cereal allergies)

- Bed-wetting

- Depression (one of the most common presenting symptoms of celiac disease)

- Diabetes, insulin-dependent (gluten, soy, and milk casein may be the primary culprits)

- Eczema (may involve both IgG and IgE antibodies at the same time)

- Epilepsy (especially when there is also a history of migraines or hyperactivity)

- Fatigue, chronic

- Fibromyalgia (biopsy of the tender spots shows IgG antibodies deposited under the skin)

- Folic acid deficiency anemia (common with celiac disease)

- Headaches (migraines, cluster)

- Inflammatory bowel disease (cow's milk enterocolitis, Crohn's disease, ulcerative colitis, and celiac disease)

- Iron-deficiency anemia

- Irritable bowel syndrome

- Middle ear disease (recurring acute or serous otitis media)

- Osteoporosis not responsive to conventional therapies (common in celiac disease)

- Rheumatoid arthritis

- Short stature

- Sleep disorders (insomnia, sleep apnea, snoring)

- Thyroid disease, underactive and overactive (common in celiac disease)

An estimated one in four people suffer from clinically significant food allergies, most of them from delayed symptoms that are probably the result of IgG food allergies. Unlike IgE allergies, IgG food allergies are very common, long lasting, and rarely self-diagnosed or treated.

And that's why the main focus of this book is to help you identify any hidden, probably IgG-based, food allergies, as well as how to get rid of or alleviate the symptoms.

UNDERSTANDING THE DIFFERENCE BETWEEN IgE AND IgG FOOD ALLERGIES

Remember the scene in the movie *Mrs. Doubtfire* where the character played by Robin Williams, out of blind jealousy, almost kills his ex-wife's allergic suitor with cayenne pepper? That was such an extreme example of an immediate-onset IgE food allergy that the cause-and-effect relationship between food and symptoms was obvious to every viewer.

As we've seen, the symptoms of a delayed-onset IgG food allergy are far more subtle and insidious, and the condition differs in a number of other ways from IgE allergies. We've summed up those differences in the following list:

- Once thought to be the only "true" food allergy, the immediate-onset type is most common in children, but rare in adults. Once thought to be uncommon at best, delayed-onset food allergy is by far the most common form of food allergy in children *and* adults.

- Allergic symptoms in immediate reactions occur within two hours of eating.

In delayed reactions, symptoms do not appear for at least two hours, not infrequently showing up twenty-four to forty-eight hours later (and there are even reports of delayed symptoms appearing three to seven days after eating).

- Immediate-onset food allergy involves one or two foods in the diet, as a rule. Delayed reactions characteristically involve three to five foods, and sometimes as many as twenty foods in very allergic individuals, who are usually found to have poor nutrition and highly "leaky" guts.

- Because a small amount of a single food is involved and the allergic symptoms appear immediately, immediate food allergy is usually self-diagnosed: you eat the food, the symptom swiftly appears, you see the connection, and you stop eating it. Due to delayed symptoms, multiple foods, and cravings for allergic foods, delayed-onset food allergies are rarely self-diagnosed, and require the skills of a health professional knowledgeable about food allergies who can run the necessary tests.

- Immediate food allergy involves foods that are rarely eaten. Delayed food allergy involves foods you may well eat every day and even crave.

- When people quit eating foods that cause immediate symptoms, they have no withdrawal or detoxification symptoms, and don't crave or miss these foods. But powerful addictive cravings and disabling withdrawal symptoms lasting for two to five days on average are reported in at least one in three people when they stop eating offending IgG foods.

- Immediate reactions to foods primarily affect the skin, airways, and digestive tract. Virtually any tissue, organ, or system of the body, including the brain, can be affected by delayed food allergy.

- Immediate food allergy can often be diagnosed with a simple skin test or blood test. Delayed reactions to food often require state-of-the-art blood tests that detect the presence of specific IgG antibodies (in the case of celiac disease, IgA antibodies as well) to foods in your blood. (We'll be discussing these tests in Chapter 7.)

If you suspect you have an IgE allergy, it's important to get yourself tested and then strictly avoid the substance in question.

Now let's take a look at the most common health problems associated with food allergy.

Chapter 3

————◄○►————

Diseases and Disorders Linked to Food Allergies

What do weight gain, eczema, and depression have in common? You may be surprised to know that they can all be symptoms of food allergy. If you're eating foods you're allergic to, your digestion, energy levels, sinuses, skin, and mental health can all suffer, as Liz's story shows.

CASE STUDY: LIZ

Diagnosed with depression at the age of fifteen, Liz spent the next two years on heavy-duty medication. Then she saw a nutritionist who found she was allergic to wheat. Once she stopped eating it, her depression lifted and she no longer needs antidepressants. However, if she has any wheat, even inadvertently in a sauce, she becomes depressed, confused, anxious, and forgetful for three to four days.

If you have any of these symptoms and they haven't responded to conventional treatment, or get better or worse when you change your diet (for instance, on holiday), then it's well worth investigating whether a hidden food allergy is involved.

INFLAMMATORY BOWEL DISEASES AND IBS

Since food allergies are triggered by immune reactions in the gut, or by a "leaky" gut that allows incompletely digested proteins from food to enter the bloodstream, it is hardly surprising that many digestive symptoms are linked to food allergy.

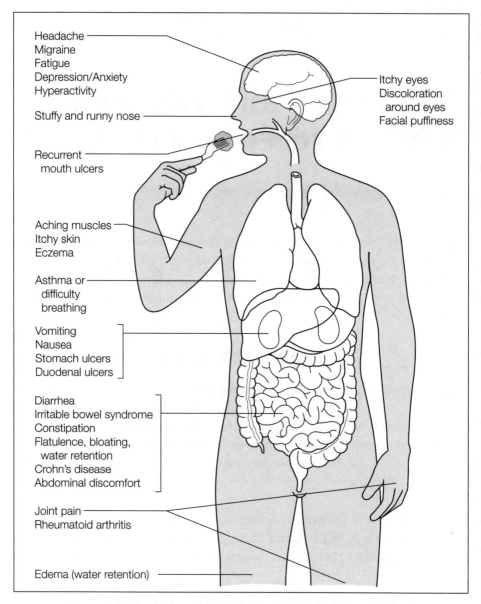

Headache
Migraine
Fatigue
Depression/Anxiety
Hyperactivity

Stuffy and runny nose

Recurrent
  mouth ulcers

Aching muscles
Itchy skin
Eczema

Asthma or
  difficulty
  breathing

Vomiting
Nausea
Stomach ulcers
Duodenal ulcers

Diarrhea
Irritable bowel syndrome
Constipation
Flatulence, bloating,
  water retention
Crohn's disease
Abdominal discomfort

Joint pain
Rheumatoid arthritis

Edema (water retention)

Itchy eyes
Discoloration
  around eyes
Facial puffiness

Figure 3.1. Common symptoms associated with food allergy.

Inflammatory Bowel Diseases

When a person bloats after eating, or experiences abdominal pain, constipation, and/or diarrhea and excessive flatulence, the first medical prerogative is to find out whether inflammation, bleeding, or ulceration is involved.

There are three common types of inflammatory bowel disease: Crohn's disease, ulcerative colitis, and celiac disease. Common symptoms for all three are pain in the joints, lack of appetite, weight loss, and fever.

In Crohn's disease, the wall of the intestine becomes sore, inflamed, and swollen. In ulcerative colitis, tiny sores form lower down in the inner lining of the colon and rectum. In addition to the symptoms mentioned above, both of these conditions are characterized by abdominal pain and cramps, diarrhea, rectal bleeding, and/or bloody stools. There are no lab tests to help identify either disease, and diagnosis is usually based on a medical history, a physical examination, and x-rays. Conventional treatment for both involves minor adjustments to the diet (for example, a decrease in fat, fiber, and lactose), anti-inflammatory drugs, and sometimes antibiotics for local infections.

Celiac disease is more than twice as common in the general population as Crohn's disease, ulcerative colitis, and cystic fibrosis combined. There are often no abdominal symptoms in the early stages. Unlike Crohn's disease and ulcerative colitis, celiac disease can be diagnosed with sophisticated lab tests and intestinal biopsies of the lining of the small intestine (more on this later). The only effective treatment is total and lifetime elimination of gluten grains from the diet, which means no wheat (including variants and hybrids such as Kamut, triticale, and spelt), rye, or barley. Oat may need to be cut out, too, although many people with celiac disease can tolerate it.

If you have inflammatory bowel disease, there's a very good chance you've got a food allergy. One study of patients with colitis found that sufferers were ten times more likely to have an IgG allergy to eggs or soy.[1] In another study, people with ulcerative colitis were more likely to react to gliadin, a protein found in gluten in wheat, rye, and barley (but not oat). Crohn's disease sufferers were also more likely to react to yeast.[2] In truth, everyone is different and it's well worth having a IgG allergy blood test if you have either of these conditions.

Irritable Bowel Syndrome (IBS)

If you have symptoms of bloating, abdominal pain, flatulence, and intermittent constipation and/or diarrhea but there's no clear evidence of inflammation, then you'll probably be diagnosed as having irritable bowel syndrome, or IBS. The most common symptom is a crampy, colicky pain or a continuous dull aching in the lower abdomen, often relieved after passing gas or having a bowel movement.

This debilitating condition wasn't really taken seriously until recently. This is illustrated by the story of Denise Lewis, one of Britain's best-known athletes, who won a gold medal for the heptathlon at the Sydney Olympics in

2000 and starred in the hit British TV show *Strictly Come Dancing*. What no one knew was that for the past thirteen years she has suffered from irritable bowel syndrome.

CASE STUDY: DENISE LEWIS

For thirteen years I've suffered from an excruciating and incurable stomach disorder called irritable bowel syndrome (IBS). At times it's left me curled up in agony, feeling as if someone was wringing out my guts by hand, and there is nothing I can do—not standing, sitting, or lying down—that can make the pain go away. Suddenly, I'll get a desperate urge to go to the bathroom and only then do I feel any relief.

I first started getting the symptoms of IBS in 1992—bloating, constipation, and gas, followed by terrible stomach pains. Like most sufferers, I wrote off the attacks as isolated incidents because they occurred months apart.

Then, in the summer of 1993, at an athletics competition in Birmingham, England, I had a particularly bad attack. It was the morning of my javelin event and the attack lasted more than two hours. I spent the run-up to the event trying every which way to get comfortable and praying for it to be over. Finally, the pain went, and somehow I managed to get out there and win. After that attack I went to my doctor, who referred me to a gastric specialist. He carried out an endoscopy. When the specialist didn't find anything, I was sent away with some anti-acid pills and a medicine to help with my constipation. They didn't really help. In essence, I was told that I just had to learn to live with it.

I started keeping a food diary to see if anything I was eating was triggering the attacks, but there seemed to be no real pattern. Then I looked at my menstrual cycle; but again there was no link.

I cut out coffee and rich foods, including my favorite ice cream, but if anything the attacks seemed more frequent. By 1998, I was having around one attack a month. Finally, in 1998, after an attack during which I vomited, I knew it was time to look for help again.

This time, I was referred to a private clinic in London's Devonshire Place, where I had an endoscopy and a colonoscopy. The doctor could see some irritation, but overall, my stomach, intestines, and bowels were pretty healthy. While he couldn't see a reason for the spasms, he was the first person to give my problem a name—irritable bowel syndrome, which was a disorder of not just the bowel but the entire intestines. He said it could be stress related, but the truth was that no one really knew why IBS occurred. I was prescribed the anti-constipation medicine again but it didn't really make any difference. At that time, I had no option but to learn to live with it. It was the run-up to the Sydney Olympics and I didn't have time to worry about being ill or in pain. I had attacks every couple of months, mostly at home in the evenings, but I just had to sweat through it and carry on with my rigorous training routine.

Then, in October last year, I heard about blood tests that could be done to establish if you were suffering from food allergies. I'd never really considered it before, because my own food diary had proved so inconclusive, but now I felt I had nothing to lose. All I had to do was prick my finger with a pin, let the blood collect in a special container and then send off the sample.

About a week later, I received the results of the tests. The report said I was very intolerant of cow's milk, moderately intolerant of yeast and egg white, and mildly intolerant of egg yolk, garlic, and cashew nuts. I wasn't surprised about the cow's milk. I regularly felt uncomfortable after drinking it, and had often drunk soy milk and eaten dairy-free products.

Since removing these foods almost a year ago I haven't had a single attack. It's not always easy to avoid the foods but the benefits are worth it for a pain-free existence. Finding out what I'm allergic to with the IgG allergy test has transformed my life. For the first time in thirteen years I'm pain-free.

Next to the common cold and chronic fatigue, IBS symptoms are the most commonly reported ailment, affecting as many as one in four people. It is most likely to appear in late teens and early adulthood and is four times more common in women than men. IBS sufferers often have a history of antibiotic use, which might actually increase the risk of developing food allergies.

If diagnosed, you might be given bran supplements, but these are rarely effective[3] and can sometimes make matters worse.[4] It's far more effective to find out which foods you're specifically allergic to, and eliminate them.

To test this approach, researchers at the University of York in the United Kingdom devised an ingenious study.[5] They tested 150 IBS sufferers using an IgG allergy test and then gave their doctors either real or fake results, and a supposedly "allergy-free" diet to follow for the next three months. Neither the patients nor their doctors knew that some of the diagnoses—and thus, the diets—were fake.

At the end of the three-month trial there was a significant improvement only in those who'd been following a diet that cut out foods they were actually allergic to. What's more, those who stuck to it most strictly had the best results. Other studies have also shown that IBS sufferers have a higher incidence of IgG allergies than non-sufferers.[6] And as IgE food allergies are not so common in IBS sufferers, it is important to test for any hidden IgG allergies.

Many people with IBS are gluten sensitive.[7-9] Some are lactose (milk sugar) intolerant. Either way, the best thing to do is to have an IgG allergy test.

WEIGHT GAIN AND WATER RETENTION

If you're carrying excess weight, chances are it could be in large part due to delayed food allergy. Rebecca's story shows how it can happen.

CASE STUDY: REBECCA

In her twenties, Rebecca's weight was stable and her skin good. She used to exercise three or four times a week. But in her thirties she started to pile on the pounds. Over three years her weight drifted from 140 pounds to over 180 pounds, and her dress size went up to 14. She also developed itchy patches on her face and had a lot of colds and sinus trouble. She didn't exercise because she didn't feel good. "I started feeling tired and lethargic and generally unwell," she said. "I didn't have the energy to go to the gym anymore."

For breakfast she'd have wheat toast, then a main meal of meat and potatoes with wheat-thickened gravy for lunch, and a sandwich for dinner. "But it seemed like the foods I ate were blowing me up, which is why I thought I could have a food allergy." She decided to test herself for a food allergy using a home test kit. The results showed she was reacting to milk, egg white, and gluten (in wheat, barley, and rye—and as in toast, gravy, and sandwiches). Within a week of excluding these foods she found that her skin and mood improved and the weight started to fall away without her consciously restricting calories. After six months she had effortlessly lost 42 pounds.

After three months of strictly avoiding the foods she'd become allergic to, she reintroduced egg whites and then milk to see if there was a reaction. Now she's fine on both foods, but still reacts to wheat.

"I can't tell you how much better I feel. I'm 100 percent," she said. "It has transformed my health. Having the food intolerance test has been the best thing I've done. I wish I'd done it sooner." In the end, she shed all the weight she'd gained during the previous three years.

Rebecca's dramatic weight gain—and loss—was unlikely to have been due solely to fat. Food allergies can cause edema, or water retention, which can also pile on the pounds. You might be holding as much as 10 pounds of extra fluid or even more without realizing it. In fact, you can easily gain up to 14 pounds in body weight this way—and lose all that in as little as forty-eight hours if you eliminate the allergen. We have observed many hundreds of overweight and obese clients lose an abundance of unsightly body fat simply by eliminating food allergens, without counting calories and often without exercising. It becomes crystal clear that there is an acceleration of fat burning associated with food-allergen elimination. Food-allergen-free diets are fat-burning diets.

CASE STUDY: MARIE

Marie was a case in point. She is allergic to wheat but insisted on eating it while on vacation in Hawaii. Her fingers swelled so much and so quickly that her marriage ring began cutting into her finger, causing bleeding. She had to have the ring cut off in an emergency room as a consequence.

How can you tell whether your weight gain is mainly fat, or substantially due to edema? Just answer the following questionnaire.

ARE YOU WATERLOGGED?

☐ Do you ever experience sudden fluctuations in your weight?

☐ Do you easily gain—and then lose—3 to 5 pounds or more in a day?

☐ Does your face look puffy, especially around and under the eyes?

☐ Do you have noticeable bags under your eyes?

☐ Does your abdomen, on pressing, feel waterlogged and bloated?

☐ Do you have to loosen your belt right after eating?

☐ Do your arms feel puffy rather than like pure fat and muscle?

☐ Do both of your ankles ever swell up?

☐ Do your fingers ever swell up so it's hard to get your rings off?

☐ Do you have dry skin or dandruff?

☐ Do you suffer from breast tenderness?

☐ Are you prone to food allergies?

If you answer "yes" to three or more of the questions above, chances are that water retention is partly to blame for your weight problem.

But a food allergy isn't the only reason for water retention. Blood sugar problems, kidney problems, heart problems, liver problems, sodium excess,

WEIGHT AND WATERLOGGING: HOW IT HAPPENS

How do food allergies lead to waterlogging? First, histamine, the stuff that makes you sneeze when it's in your nose, makes tiny blood vessels called capillaries leakier. This allows the immune system's army of white blood cells to move into the battlefield—your tissues. At the same time, plenty of fluid accompanying the white blood cells passes into your tissues, where it's retained for days, even weeks. If this is happening several times a day, you literally become waterlogged.

Allergic reactions also mess up the balance of prostaglandins, hormone-like substances made from essential fats, and this, too, can lead to water retention as well as abdominal bloating. Take the case of Joanne M. (see case study). She didn't just have weight to lose, but girth.

As previously stated, there's much more to the weight gain than water. One of the prostaglandins released during inflammation and allergic reactions, prostaglandin E2 (PGE2), dramatically slows down fat metabolism, so that fat becomes much easier to store in cells than to burn off once stored. Also, the more frequent your allergic reactions, the more resistant you become to insulin, the hormone that keeps your blood sugar in balance. This is because the body releases masses of immune messengers called cytokines to deal with the allergy, and cytokines make you less responsive to insulin. Also, repeated allergic reactions mean that more garbage—that is, immune complexes—ends up in your bloodstream as your immune cells struggle, often unsuccessfully, to fight off the invaders.

It's up to your liver, your body's detoxifying organ, to clean up the ensuing mess. But eventually, your liver's detox capacity will get overloaded (sometimes, as in celiac disease, your liver actually becomes injured and damaged by eating gluten). When this happens, your body dumps the toxins in the least harmful place—your fat cells. The more intoxicated your fat cells become—and the higher to PGE2 released by allergic reactions—the slower the body's ability to metabolize fat, and the more fat is retained; and the more weight you gain, the harder it becomes to shift those extra pounds. This is why people with allergies can find it harder and harder to lose weight. Also, this continual process of inhibition of fat metabolism and overintoxication can turn a mild food allergy into something more severe. It also invariably leads to chronic fatigue.

and essential fat deficiency can also promote watery weight gain. Here's what you can do to rule these out:

- Avoid sugary or refined foods and stimulants such as coffee.

- Eat five to nine servings of a variety of fruits and vegetables every day (one serving is one-half to one full cup).

- Eat nuts and seeds (rich in essential fats, plus magnesium and potassium).

- Eat whole foods and nonallergic whole grains such as beans, lentils, brown rice, and whole-grain bread (be aware that you may be gluten sensitive and have to avoid whole wheat, rye, and barley).

- Eat more oily fish such as salmon, halibut, orange roughy, and sardines (all rich in essential fats) in unfried and unbreaded form, and less meat.

- Don't add salt to your food, unless it's low-sodium salt.

- Choose "low sodium" processed foods.

- Drink the equivalent of eight glasses of water, including herbal teas, a day.

This way of eating alone may cause you to rapidly lose weight if water retention is part of your problem. But if you are finding it hard to shift weight, the most important thing is to find out which foods you are allergic to and stay off them.

CASE STUDY: JOANNE M.

I used to stand in front of the mirror, grab a handful of my stomach—and despair. After a big meal I looked five months pregnant! It wasn't just my weight, which hovered around 154 pounds, it was the bloating (I'd gone up to a size 14) and the physical symptoms. I'd have to undo my trousers every time I had a big meal and I was often constipated.

When I was in my late teens, I was diagnosed with IBS. Instead of looking for the cause, doctors simply prescribed drugs to ease the symptoms. Reading up about the problem, I got the impression a high-fiber diet would help the constipation and stop my stomach from bloating. But my health regimen of whole wheat bread, baked potatoes, and beans was actually making it worse.

I felt exhausted all the time and usually fell asleep by 9:30 in the evening. My husband, Steve, kept telling me I had to do something about it. So in September 2002 I sent away for a food intolerance blood test. The results told me I was sensitive to all dairy products, yeast, salmon, trout, haricot beans, and string beans. Within a week I was going to the bathroom every two days (instead of weekly), my stomach bloating was gone, and I was down to a size 10. My lethargy was caused by the yeasty foods I ate. I've gone down to 129 pounds and look so much trimmer now.

FATIGUE, INSOMNIA, AND SNORING

Fatigue is the reason for so many doctors' visits that a new term has been coined—TATT ("tired all the time"). More than half of people diagnosed with chronic fatigue syndrome (CFS) also have allergies to foods, airborne substances, and drugs, according to one scientific review.[10] Another study reports that about 50 percent of CFS patients have "nonallergic rhinitis," meaning they have nasal symptoms that are unrelated to an IgE immediate-onset allergy.[11] More often than not, these symptoms are caused or aggravated by IgG food allergies.

If you're having trouble falling asleep, waking up frequently during the night, waking up early and not being able to get back to sleep, waking up tired and/or depressed, and/or snoring loudly when you sleep, food allergy might be contributing. Food allergies are certainly not the only reasons for fatigue and insomnia but if you are tired all the time or unable to sleep or both, and haven't been able to identify a cause, then getting tested for a food allergy is a very sensible route to follow.

HEADACHES AND MIGRAINES

Frequent headaches or migraines are extremely debilitating. One migraine sufferer put it this way: "When I had headaches, I only lived half a life. When I had a migraine, everything else was obliterated by the pain—my family, my work, my name. I was living half my life on another planet, a planet of torture and pain."

Migraines are thought to happen when arteries in the scalp dilate, and those in the brain constrict. Aside from the pain, they may involve visual disturbances, nausea, vomiting, and sensitivity to light and noise. It's an exhausting experience, and the sufferer usually has to sleep it off afterward. They affect more women than men, and about one in ten people.

A cluster headache is the most severe of all headaches, found more often in men than women. It often comes on during sleep and/or twenty to forty minutes after drinking alcohol. Sufferers will experience severe pain, usually behind one eye, described as feeling like a red-hot poker being driven into the eye socket. They can last for hours or even days nonstop, often occur in batches on a daily basis, and can also bring on symptoms such as tearing in the affected eye; a stuffed-up nose; feeling hot; a sweaty face, neck, and trunk; nausea, vomiting, and/or diarrhea; a drop in blood pressure; and even heart arrhythmia. Unsurprisingly, they're incapacitating and can drive sufferers to the brink of their endurance. Some cluster headache sufferers seriously consider suicide as an option.

While the trigger of both migraines and cluster headaches is still largely unknown, there is growing evidence that in many cases food allergy is the culprit. About a quarter of migraine patients report that their symptoms can be initiated by certain foods.[12] One double-blind study on forty children with migraines reported a decrease or complete elimination of attacks in over 80 percent of children who avoided some foods. Associated symptoms also improved, including abdominal pain, seizures, asthma, "growing pains," and eczema.[13] Other studies have observed a decrease in the number of attacks in 80 percent of patients on avoidance diets.[14-15] We believe that testing and eliminating food allergens should be the first avenue of attack on migraine and cluster headaches, not the last.

CASE STUDY: ALISON

Alison suffered increasingly severe headaches and migraines for ten years. Often the headaches would be accompanied by sickness and flashing lights, and she would have to retreat into a darkened room to rest for a day and two nights. She also suffered from a "fuzzy" head and felt very lethargic. She also suffered from the pain of arthritis and sinusitis.

Since doctors could not offer a solution other than painkillers to help ease the pain, she had an IgG food allergy test. The results showed an intolerance to dairy products, yeast, seafood, and nuts.

Within a couple of days of cutting these foods out of her diet, she began to feel better. Her head felt clearer, her energy levels improved, and her symptoms of sinusitis and rheumatoid arthritis also eased considerably. The number of migraines she had dropped dramatically. Recently, she ate half a cheese sandwich—and rediscovered the importance of sticking to her avoidance diet. "By the end of the afternoon, I could feel a headache coming on," she said. "It was bad the next day and only eased off the day after that."

In our experience, the majority of migraine and cluster headaches can be traced to delayed-onset food allergy. The most common allergic villains in migraines and headaches (and there's often more than one) are cow's milk, eggs, wheat, oranges, benzoic acid (interacts with vitamin C in soft drinks to produce benzene, a known carcinogen), cheese, and chemical additives, especially tartrazine (FD&C Yellow No. 5) and MSG. Typically, the average time lag between eating an offending food and developing a headache or migraine is forty-eight hours, which makes it much harder to self-diagnose. As the food allergy implicated in migraines is almost always delayed-onset, we recommend an IgG allergy test.

ARTHRITIS AND JOINT PAIN

Arthritis is a debilitating disease that affects nine out of ten people by the age of sixty. There are two main kinds—osteoarthritis and rheumatoid arthritis. The most common is osteoarthritis, affecting joints that have been injured or simply worn out, often through inadequate nutrition, poor posture, and lack of mobility, which is necessary to keep joints flexible and healthy. It usually comes on after age fifty.

Rheumatoid arthritis, however, can strike at any age and affects about 1 in 100 people, mostly women. This is a very destructive inflammatory disease that causes pain, swelling, stiffness, and loss of function in the joints, and can also affect other parts of the body. It is also an autoimmune condition; that is, there is evidence that the body's own immune system attacks the joints. People with the disease may experience chronic fatigue, occasional fever, and a general sense of malaise. It can be mild or severe and active most of the time, last for many years, and lead to serious joint damage and disability. It is so disabling that half of patients have to stop working within ten years of diagnosis.

No conventional treatment can cure or reverse rheumatoid arthritis, but there are medications that can relieve its symptoms and slow or halt its progress. They include nonsteroidal anti-inflammatory drugs such as ibuprofen or Aleve (to help relieve pain and inflammation), corticosteroids (to reduce inflammation and slow joint damage), and disease-modifying antirheumatic drugs (to slow or halt the progression of rheumatoid arthritis). Each of these treatments has many side effects—stomach upset, stomach ulcers with bleeding, "leaky gut" lining, esophageal reflux, easy bruising, thinning of bones, cataracts, weight gain, diabetes, kidney damage, high blood pressure, blurry vision, and increased susceptibility to infection. There is also evidence that after about ten years on these medications, they cause an acceleration of joint tissue degeneration and joint instability following surgical joint replacement.

With rheumatoid arthritis, as with other autoimmune diseases like lupus or type 1 diabetes, it's well worth suspecting food allergy as the trigger—especially gluten, soy, and/or dairy sensitivities. Our twenty-five years of clinical experience have taught us that rheumatoid arthritis is frequently caused or provoked by food allergy, and that most rheumatoid arthritics under the age of seventy respond dramatically to food allergy elimination, together with an optimum nutrition diet and supplements, including natural anti-inflammatory nutrients and herbs such as omega-3 fish oil, curcumin, *Boswellia,* and hop extracts, to name a few. (See Patrick's book *Say No to Arthritis* for a comprehensive nutrition-based strategy.)

One theory about why food allergy could trigger autoimmune conditions is that the immune system could become sensitive to a food protein such as soy or milk protein, and wrongly "cross-react" to tissue in the body with similar, difficult to distinguish protein. While an allergy-free diet doesn't help everybody, studies do show that some people experience great benefits. In one study, 9 percent of a group of rheumatoid arthritis patients improved when put on an allergy-free diet, and worsened when taken off it. To make sure these results were real, six of these patients were reintroduced to small amounts of nonallergic foods or allergic foods without their knowing which they were taking. Four got noticeably worse on the allergy food, not the placebo.[16]

CASE STUDY: CATHY

In November, Cathy heard Dr. Braly speak on the radio and remarked, "You could have been speaking directly to me, so specific were your descriptions of my medical problem."

In December the laboratory technician came to her Ohio home to draw her blood. Thirteen days later she received her food allergy test results showing evidence of delayed food allergy to wheat, cheese, eggs, yeast, and bananas. Late in December she stopped eating all these foods. "I don't respond well to change and the first days off these foods I had a terrible 'killer headache' [withdrawal headache] that disappeared on the fourth day as quickly as it appeared on the first day of food avoidance. Gradually my symptoms began to abate and each day was a little better." Within one week she definitely felt better and within two weeks the arthritic pains had subsided to the point that she could now sleep in her favorite position, lying on her (formerly arthritic) left elbow. During this time she went with her husband to her favorite restaurant where she ordered "a normal meal of pasta [wheat]." The very next day the pain and other symptoms she had forgotten returned. "This helped to confirm in my mind how much my body really needed these changes."

Seven weeks after eliminating allergic foods from her diet, Cathy reported the following: She was basically free of joint swelling and pain, back pain, and the pains down her arms and legs. Her energy level was back to normal. The edema (fluid retention) was gone. Cathy had lost 15 pounds since Christmas, the first 10 pounds in the first week or so. The heartburn and heart palpitations had disappeared. The skin rash and itching was gone. Her sleeping pattern was again back to normal. And, Cathy was off all medications, including all anti-inflammatory drugs!

CASE STUDY: JOHN

John developed both psoriasis and arthritis in his toes, fingers, ankles, and knees at the age of twenty-three. By age forty he couldn't sleep at night from the pain and had to go upstairs on hands and knees. Walking just 100 yards was painful. Holidays were awful. He used to have to think carefully where to park the car when going out so as not to have to walk too far. He saw consultants, read books, and took lots of medication, which controlled the pain but had their own side effects—stomach pain and depression. Sometimes he had steroid injections to make the pain subside, but it would return later in the day.

Then John heard about food allergy testing. Although his doctor actively discouraged testing of that type, saying that there was "absolutely no clinical evidence" that altering diet would improve such a condition, John went ahead and discovered he was allergic to three different foods. He was shocked to discover that the main one was white fish, as everyone had been saying to cut out red meat and eat much more white and oily fish. (Fish is an excellent food—unless you are allergic to it.) Egg white was another—and the last was tea.

John cut them all out. Gradually the number of painkillers he needed lessened and eventually he stopped completely. In his own words, "Life is now pain- and tablet-free and I have complete mobility. I am amazed at the difference in my quality of life simply by making such simple adjustments."

While food allergy isn't the only factor contributing to arthritis, we recommend exploring it if you do suffer from arthritis or joint aches and pains.

ECZEMA AND OTHER SKIN PROBLEMS

Eczema can vary from mild to severe. In mild forms the skin is dry, hot, and itchy, while in more severe forms the skin can become broken, raw, and bleeding, often leaving a trail of dead skin on clothes, carpets, and chairs. Conventional treatment involves anti-inflammatory skin creams—usually some form of cortisone. This reduces the severity but the skin remains sensitive to flare-ups.

The causes of eczema are many and varied, and depend on the particular type a person has. Atopic eczema is thought to be a hereditary condition, and is diagnosed if the affected person has other allergic symptoms and/or a family history of such conditions, including asthma and hay fever. It is highly likely that a person with this form of eczema has food and possibly chemical and/or inhalant allergies. Other types of eczema are caused by irritants such as chemicals and detergents, allergens such as nickel, and yeast growths. In later years eczema can be caused by a circulatory problem in the legs. The causes of other types of eczema remain to be explained, though links with environmental factors and stress are being explored.

The most common food allergy that can provoke eczema, especially in children, is milk. IgG antibodies to milk have been found to be much more common in both children and adults with eczema.[17-21] Other investigators have also found IgG sensitivity to eggs to be far more common in eczema sufferers.[22] Despite overwhelming evidence of an association with hidden IgG food allergy, very few eczema sufferers are tested for IgG delayed food allergy by their doctors.

CASE STUDY: LIZA

Liza is a case in point. She had suffered from eczema, and had used a cortisone cream and other steroid-based creams, all her life. Her eczema was worst on her hands and arms. She had been to an herbalist who charged her hundreds of dollars to carry out so-called allergy tests. He used an electronic machine "that looked like it was out of the 1950s," placing it on the palm of her hand and then listening to the beeps the machine made. He claimed that the noises determined her food sensitivities. He told her to cut out a long list of foods and also recommended that she take thirteen tablets a day.

(Be skeptical of these exotic, unproven "food allergy tests," including the very popular "muscle testing" technique used by many alternative health professionals today. Be especially wary if they place the tested food in a small bottle or vial in your hand or somewhere on your skin, and not in your mouth. In one well-publicized study, three different chiropractors, each using the same muscle-testing technique on the same patient, disagreed with one another by identifying entirely different allergic foods.)

Liza did manage to stick to the diet—and her eczema got so bad that her skin blistered. After four days her eczema was worse than ever and it took another two and a half weeks for it to improve at all. Not surprisingly, she didn't stick with the diet for long.

We tested her using a proper IgG food allergy blood test and found she was strongly allergic to dairy products and mildly sensitive to gluten and egg white. She was also given a vitamin A–based skin cream. This can help to keep the skin healthy once the inflammation calms down.

In her case, stress made her skin worse and, noticing that she often had several cups of coffee and a couple of Red Bull drinks each day, we recommended she cut out any source of caffeine. (Both stress and caffeine put extraordinary strain on one's stress glands, the adrenals, leading to adrenal fatigue and increased inflammation.)

One month later this is what she said: "I feel so much better. Nothing like as tired. I have one coffee a week, no headaches, no side effects. No bloating. The milk avoidance itself wasn't so difficult. But I was amazed to find out how many foods had hidden milk so it took a week to discover what I could and couldn't have. Overall, it's been fine. It's not as hard as it used to be at the beginning. My skin is a lot better. I have no sores and no cuts—it's just a little dry. The vitamin A cream really works very well. I have lost a couple of pounds. I am really surprised how easy I found it to cut out the caffeine, and I have more energy, not less."

Three months later Liza is still eczema-free and has not had to use the cortisone cream once since she went on her allergy-free diet.

While food allergy is clearly not the only cause of skin problems such as eczema, we believe anyone with eczema, and also conditions like hives and dermatitis, should strongly consider having an IgG food allergy test. In more cases than not, an allergy-free diet makes a big difference.

ASTHMA AND NASAL AND SINUS PROBLEMS

Some of the most common food allergy symptoms are constant coughing, sniffling and snuffling, excessive mucus formation, and a blocked nose. This can lead to or be associated with a variety of diseases of the airways, such as asthma, bronchitis, rhinitis (hay fever), and sinusitis. The most serious and life-threatening of these is undoubtedly asthma. According to a May 2001 report by the World Health Organization (WHO), 100 to 150 million people around the world are asthmatic and the number is growing by 50 percent every decade, killing at least 180,000 people each year.

"Seventeen million Americans suffer from asthma today, 5 million of whom are children, and some 29 million Americans will suffer from asthma by 2020," predicts the nonprofit Pew Environmental Health Commission. Asthma kills 5,000 Americans a year and hospitalizes 500,000. The elderly and children, especially black children, are at greatest risk (see Chapter 4 for a discussion of childhood asthma).

Asthma is commonly an allergic condition because allergens stimulate the release of histamine and leukotrienes, chemical mediators, from sensitized immune cells lining the airways. This causes the airway tubes to become highly irritated and very sensitive. When this happens the tissue in the tubes becomes swollen, and gelatin-like mucus begins to plug up the air passages.

The result is potentially serious bouts of wheezing, and coughing (easily provoked by laughing, exercising, crying, or breathing cold air). This may lead on to other symptoms—shortness of breath, pressure in the chest, and difficult breathing or "tight throat"—which can make asthmatics feel as if they are slowly suffocating to death. Irritable, hypersensitive, swollen airways are very prone to going into spasms. When this happens, it is called an asthma attack.

An attack may last for a few hours or go on for weeks, and may never get past the wheezing and coughing stage, or may require all a sufferer's energy to keep breathing. Frequent visits to the emergency room, sometimes resulting in hospitalization, happen during these very stressful, frightening times.

Why is this debilitating disorder becoming more widespread and dangerous? The reasons are many: the declining quality of our diets with associated nutrient and phytonutrient deficiencies, stressful or inactive lifestyles, poor quality of sleep, increasing exposure to airborne and food allergens, increased incidence of other allergic conditions (otitis, sinusitis, eczema, hives, and a family history of atopic allergies occur more frequently in asthmatics), chemicals and toxins in our environment, overuse of aspirin and aspirin substitutes, sulfites in white wine as well as dried fruits and other processed foods, and an overdependence on inhalers.

In mainstream medicine until recently, the assumption dictating therapy was that asthma was basically an airway-narrowing disease. Consequently, medication to dilate or enlarge the airways is the norm, and so-called inhaled corticosteroids have also been thrown into the mix.

The problems with this approach are threefold: when used excessively (more than a canister and a half per month), inhalers are associated with a dramatic increase in death rates. Long-term use of inhaled corticosteroids doesn't seem to change the progression of the disease, merely controls symptoms, and has other adverse effects in children. What's more, the conventional wisdom that inhalers should be used regularly has been overturned by research that shows you are better off using them as and when you need them (and as little as possible) than having this constant intake of steroids.[23]

A better and more lasting approach to treating asthma—and many nasal or sinus problems—is to address the underlying causes of airway inflammation and hyperirritability, not just the short-term relief of wheezing, coughing, and shortness of breath. This begins with the identification and elimination of air-borne and food allergens. The top suspects are wheat, milk, and eggs,[24] while colorings, preservatives (especially sulfites), and other chemical food additives may also be implicated, along with dust mites, mold, animal dander, and cock-roach antigens (proteins from the insects' saliva, eggs, and so on).

As you'll see in Chapter 8, improving nutrition will dramatically strength-en the immune system and reduce allergic reactions. Also, there are many excellent natural anti-inflammatory herbs and nutrients that can make an asth-matic less dependent on inhalers. Among these are quercetin (see page 101) and butterbur. A recent trial by the University of Heidelberg in Germany, involving eighty adults and children suffering from asthma, found that 40 per-cent could reduce their use of medication by taking a daily supplement of butterbur root.[25]

LOW MOODS, "BRAIN FOGS," AND DEPRESSION

Most people don't think of food allergies as a potential cause of low mood, chronic depression, poor concentration, anxiety, or even more severe condi-tions such as schizophrenia. Yet the knowledge that allergy to foods and chem-icals can adversely affect moods, cognition, and behavior in susceptible individuals has been known for a very long time. Food allergies have been proven to cause a diverse range of symptoms including chronic fatigue, "brain fog," slowed thought processes, lack of motivation, irritability, agitation, aggres-sive behavior, nervousness, anxiety, depression, alcoholism and substance abuse, schizophrenia, hyperactivity (ADHD), panic attacks, autism, and varied learning disabilities.[26-35] We'll discuss the link to problems in children in detail in the next chapter.

A doctor from Germany, Dr. Joseph Egger, was one of the first pioneers studying the link between allergy and mental health. He decided to test thirty patients suffering from anxiety, depression, confusion, or difficulty in concen-trating for allergy, using a double-blind placebo-controlled trial, by giving the patients either dummy foods, or their allergenic foods, in small quantities, dis-guised so they didn't know what they were eating. The results showed that the food allergens alone were able to produce severe depression, nervousness, feeling of anger without a particular object, loss of motivation, and severe men-tal blankness. Not surprisingly, the foods that produced most severe mental reactions were the common food allergens wheat, milk, cane sugar, and eggs.[36]

Another pioneer of food and chemical sensitivity was Dr. Benjamin Feingold, whose Feingold Diet became famous in the 1970s. He investigated the possibility of food allergies and sensitivity to salicylates (such as aspirin) in ninety-six patients diagnosed as suffering from alcohol dependency, major depressive disorders, and schizophrenia, compared to sixty-two control subjects selected from adult hospital staff members for a possible food/chemical intolerance.

The results showed that the group of patients diagnosed as depressives had the highest number of allergies: 80 percent were allergic to barley, and all were allergic to egg white. Over half the alcoholics tested were found to be allergic to egg white, milk, rye, and barley (similar to the food allergens affecting alcoholics identified by Dr. Joan Mathews Larson in her pathbreaking book *Seven Weeks to Sobriety*—more on food allergies and alcoholism in Chapter 5). Of the people with schizophrenia, 80 percent were found to be allergic to both milk and eggs. Only 9 percent of the control group were found to suffer from any allergies.[37]

These studies are prime examples of how problems created by allergies can often produce a multitude of mental and emotional as well as physical symptoms, because they affect brain chemistry and function, and even the whole body. The state of inflammation and neurochemical changes induced by an allergic reaction is found in many mental health conditions, from depression to autism to attention deficit hyperactivity disorder (ADHD), and is probably one of the main mechanisms by which a food allergy affects the brain. What's more, food allergies are very specific to the individual, as are the symptoms they create, so any diagnosis can only be made individually by proper food allergy testing.

When tested in a clinical laboratory that properly maintains a consistently high degree of quality control, it is not at all uncommon to find that putting a person on the allergy-free diet they need relieves symptoms of depression, insomnia, daytime drowsiness, anxiety, panic attacks, hyperactivity, irritability, outbursts of anger, and on occasion even schizophrenia. So if you suffer from poor concentration, insomnia, depression, anxiety, or other symptoms of depleted mental health, it's well worth investigating whether food allergies play a part. If you would like to further explore the role that nutrition and food allergy plays in alcoholism, substance abuse, compulsive overeating, depression, anxiety, and/or insomnia, please contact the addiction treatment centers listed in Resources (also see Chapter 5).

Chapter 4

—◁◦▷—

Children
and Food Allergies

O f all people, children show most clearly that our twenty-first-century diets and lifestyles are resulting in more and more food allergies and sensitivities. And along with those allergies go a wide range of childhood illnesses and other conditions—from middle ear disease to attention deficit hyperactive disorder (ADHD). Let's look at these now.

THE ADHD EPIDEMIC

ADHD is fast becoming a household name in America. In 1990, 750,000 American children were diagnosed with it. Today, that figure is estimated to be over 4 million, of which about 3 million kids have been diagnosed. In Britain it is vastly underdiagnosed, yet the symptoms are estimated to occur in a quarter of a million children under the age of seventeen.

ADHD affects five times as many boys as girls. A third or more ADHD children will grow up to be ADHD adults. There is no laboratory or clinical test available yet that definitively diagnoses the condition; a diagnosis is based on observations of inattention, hyperactivity, and impulsivity so serious they impair a child's ability to function. Many children with ADHD take stimulant medications under a doctor's prescription—usually amphetamine-like drugs Ritalin and Concerta, or a "cocktail" of amphetamines called Adderall—to help them pay attention, calm down, and perform better in school. The short-term effectiveness of these medications in reducing hyperactivity and improving concentration and learning is about 60 to 70 percent.

Largely ignored, however, is the role that food allergy and chemical-food-additive sensitivities play in children with ADHD. In a classic study by Dr. Joseph Egger and colleagues at the University of Munich in Germany, seventy-six children with severe ADHD were kept on a strict hypoallergenic (very low allergic potential) diet for four weeks.[1] The results were amazing: 82 percent of the children got better on the hypoallergenic diet. One out of four children with severe ADHD recovered completely. Even more remarkably, most of the other non-ADHD symptoms improved with the diet, as well. Table 4.1 shows what happened.

	NUMBER OF CHILDREN SUFFERING FROM IT	
SYMPTOM	BEFORE DIET CHANGE	ON DIET
Antisocial behavior	32	13
Headaches	48	9
Seizures/fits	14	1
Abdominal pain or discomfort	54	8
Chronic rhinitis (nonseasonal)	33	9
Leg aches ("growing pains")	33	6
Skin rashes	28	9
Mouth ulcers (aphthous ulcers/canker sores)	15	5
Emotional problems (depression, anxiety, etc.)	7	0

TABLE 4.1. RESULTS OF DR. JOSEPH EGGER'S STUDY

Egger then gave the children foods with artificial food colors and preservatives. He found the most problematic common substances were the chemical additives tartrazine (FD&C Yellow No. 5) and benzoic acid. However, no child reacted to these two food additives alone. A total of forty-six different foods provoked allergic symptoms. Soy, cow's milk, wheat, grapes, chocolate, oranges, eggs, and peanuts were the most common food allergens. Foods that did not cause symptoms included cabbage, lettuces, cauliflower, celery—and duck eggs!

Having identified which foods each child was allergic to, Egger then ran a test, giving the children either a placebo or a tiny amount of the food allergen without either the child or the researcher knowing which was given (in other words, a placebo-controlled double-blind test). This showed these children definitely were reacting to specific foods and chemicals.

In the United Kingdom, the leading child psychiatrist Professor Eric Taylor was somewhat skeptical about the reports he was getting from parents saying their children were behaving better on diets excluding chemical additives and/or common food allergens. He decided to investigate with another double-blind trial.[2] He took seventy-eight hyperactive children and placed them on a "few foods" elimination diet. Fifty-nine of the children showed improved behavior during the trial. For nineteen of these children it was possible to disguise foods or additives, or both, that reliably provoked behavioral problems by mixing them with other tolerated foods and to test their effect in a placebo-controlled double-blind design. The results of this trial on these nineteen children showed that the provoking foods did worsen ratings of behavior and impair psychological test performance.

Carrie's story shows how dramatic the improvement can be.

CASE STUDY: CARRIE

From the age of two, Carrie had suffered from extreme hyperactivity, chronic insomnia, irritability, headaches, frequent sinus and middle ear infections, and joint pains, and had dark circles under her eyes. None of the treatments and tests that she underwent brought her any relief. When Carrie was five, her parents had her tested for IgG food allergy. They found their daughter was allergic to twenty-two different foods. She was also found to have a number of airborne allergies—to mold, house-dust mites, pollens, and dog dander. Taking all twenty-two foods out of her diet and removing some of the sources of airborne allergens from her home improved her symptoms very quickly. At ten years old, Carrie is very well, with none of her previous symptoms.

AUTISM

Among autistic children the evidence for food allergy, especially allergy to gluten grains and milk, is even higher than for children with ADHD. Much of the impetus for recognizing the importance of dietary intervention has come from parents who have noticed vast improvements in their autistic children after changing their diets.

Wheat and dairy products—and the highly allergic proteins they contain, gluten and casein—are the foods linked most strongly to autism. These proteins are difficult to digest and, especially if introduced too early in life, may result in an allergy. Fragments of both gluten and casein (more specifically gluteomorphin from gluten and casomorphin from casein), known as peptides, can mimic chemicals in the brain called endorphins, so they're often referred to as "exomorphins."

By mimicking the body's own morphine-like endorphins, exomorphins cause the body to become less sensitive to its own natural endorphins, which leads to cravings for even more of these exomorphins found in milk and wheat.[3]

The most common food allergies and chemical intolerances in autistic children are as follows:

- Wheat and other gluten-containing grains

- Milk and other dairy products containing casein

- Citrus fruits

- Chocolate

- Salicylates (as in aspirin)

- Foods in the nightshade family (potatoes, tomatoes, eggplants, peppers)

- Acetaminophen (Tylenol, for example)

- Tartrazine, benzoic acid, and monosodium glutamate (MSG)

If you have a child with autism or Asperger's syndrome, we strongly recommend you investigate food allergy as a contributory cause. If you'd like to find out more about the nutritional approach to autism, see Patrick's book *Optimum Nutrition for the Mind* (Basic Health Publications, 2004).

EAR, NOSE, AND THROAT INFECTIONS

Almost every parent is aware of the agony their child experiences with recurring ear infections, which can often involve the nose and throat as well. The most common and serious is middle ear infection, of which there are two types: acute otitis media, and otitis media with effusion (also called serous otitis media, and nicknamed "glue ear"), which involves fluid buildup in the middle ear.

Signs and symptoms of acute otitis media include:

- Severe and persistent pain in one or both ears

- Ear tugging or pulling

- Fever up to 104°F (fever with chills or fever with a headache may be a sign of more serious complications)

- Irritability, lethargy

- Loss of appetite, nausea, vomiting and/or diarrhea, and concurrent signs of allergic rhinitis (frequent sneezing, runny or congested nose, nose rubbing, eye burning), catarrh, and recurrent tonsillitis may also appear in as many as 80 percent of otitis media sufferers.

In otitis media with effusion, the signs and symptoms are:

• Ear discomfort (ear popping, ear pressure, earache, hearing loss)

• Behavioral or emotional changes (poor sleeping, irritability, underachieving in school, many of the signs and symptoms of ADHD), and speech or language problems

More often than not, the immediate "solution" is antibiotics,[4-6] despite the well-published evidence that the routine, repetitive use of antibiotics in treating otitis media increases its recurrence three to sixfold. Eighty percent or more of this epidemic of ear problems could be avoided simply by identifying and avoiding food allergens, as at least four out of five of these children are food allergic.

What happens is this: the allergic reactions cause the Eustachian tube that drains the middle ear to swell and close. Identify and stop eating allergic foods, and the Eustachian tube will open and drain, and infection and/or fluid buildup will disappear. No more monthly visits to the doctor's office, or prescriptions for antibiotics that don't work very well. It's that simple.

In our opinion, every single child suffering from repeated bouts of otitis media should be tested and treated for delayed-onset IgG food allergy.

ASTHMA

As we saw in the preceding chapter, food allergies often result in diseases of the airways, the most serious of which is asthma.[7] Of the 17 million Americans who suffer from asthma today, 5 million are children. In the United Kingdom, one in five children now have asthma, compared to just one in twenty-five adults—in fact, asthma is now the leading cause of school absenteeism for children under fifteen years old.

We've shown how allergic reactions can cause the airways to become irritated or to constrict, leading to a cascade of symptoms that can have sufferers wheezing, coughing, or even fighting to breathe. In children, this can be a real blow to their confidence and leave them in fear of the next attack. But an overreliance on inhalers, as we've seen, isn't the answer. They can be a huge health risk—and if corticosteroids are involved, your child's growth in height can actually be slowed by about an inch a year.

Trying to treat the wheezing and coughing rather than the underlying cause is too limited a solution. We recommend that every child with asthma be checked for IgG food allergy.

SLEEPING PROBLEMS

Many parents struggle to get their child to sleep, not realizing that food allergies may be making them hyperactive. That glass of milk or piece of toast before bed may make matters worse, not better.

A study of seventy-one babies, fifty of them poor sleepers, showed that milk is a common allergen in infants. The babies with sleep problems showed raised levels of IgG antibodies to milk, and when milk was eliminated from their diets, their sleep pattern became normal. When milk was then reintroduced to their diets, their sleeplessness returned.[8] In another study, seventeen under-fives were referred to a sleep clinic for their continual waking and crying during sleep times. To determine if a food allergy could be contributing to their insomnia, cow's milk was excluded from their diets. Within six weeks, the children were falling asleep more easily, and slept more solidly and for longer—sleeping, on average, from five and a half to thirteen hours. Reintroducing cow's milk into their diets caused their insomnia to recur.[9]

There can, of course, be other allergies behind sleeplessness, so the best course of action is to have your child tested.

BED-WETTING

Bed-wetting is another problem for families with young children—tens of thousands of them, in fact. Between 10 and 15 percent of children wet their beds regularly, and 5 percent of them will still have the problem in adulthood.

Bed-wetting children can be consumed by feelings of guilt and low self-esteem as they see how ever-present piles of laundry and odors of urine affect their parents. Bed-wetters are often reluctant to stay overnight with friends, or engage in a number of activities children normally do. And there can be related problems. ADHD—commonly a food allergic condition—is more prevalent in bed-wetters.[10] So on top of the bed-wetting, many children with the condition have to cope with a range of typical ADHD symptoms (see page 39).

In the early 1990s Dr. Joseph Egger—then at London's Great Ormond Street Hospital for Sick Children—studied twenty-one children with migraines or hyperactivity who were also bed-wetters, and who had previously responded well to a "few foods" diet (a diet free from the common allergenic foods). He identified which of the foods provoked migraines or hyperactivity in each child and removed these from their diets. The bed-wetting stopped altogether in over half the children and decreased in a further fifth of them.[11]

In our experience, most bed-wetters have hidden food allergies. Allergic reactions can irritate the bladder wall, and as we've seen, also provoke sleep disorders—of which bed-wetting is one. When the food allergy is solved, the child sleeps more restfully, and is able to wake up to make it to the toilet in time.

TYPE 1 DIABETES

Diabetes is a chronic disease in which the human body either doesn't produce enough insulin—the hormone that helps regulate blood sugar and turn it into energy—or is unable to use it properly. The high levels of sugar in a diabetic's blood mean he or she has low energy.

There are two primary types of diabetes. About 90 percent of diabetics have type 2, which used to be called "adult-onset" diabetes because it usually sets in in adulthood. Type 1 diabetes is usually detected in childhood. People with type 1 produce very little or no insulin, and need daily injections of the hormone to prevent their blood sugar levels from getting dangerously high. Hence its other name, "insulin-dependent" diabetes. An estimated 16 million Americans have either type 1 or type 2 diabetes—and about 5.4 million of these diabetics have yet to be diagnosed. Each year 625,000 new cases of type 2 diabetes are diagnosed. Type 1 diabetes affects about 1 million Americans, with 30,000 new cases diagnosed each year. Both types of diabetes are more common among Native Americans, Hispanics, and African Americans.

Type 1 diabetes tends to run in families, suggesting a genetic predisposition to developing it. But its cause is still unknown. So what's the link with food allergy?

In this kind of diabetes, the child's immune system attacks and eventually destroys insulin-producing cells in the pancreas. It is therefore classed as an "autoimmune" disease. There is increasing evidence that what might be happening is that the child becomes allergic to a particular food protein, and that the immune system reacts not only to this, but to a similar protein in the pancreas. This "cross-reaction" theory is gaining credence and suggests that, in children who may be genetically susceptible to developing the condition, the major trigger might be introducing allergy-provoking foods too early—before the gut and immune system are fully mature.[12-20]

These so-called diabetogenic foods, in order of importance, include:

- Gluten grains
- Soy products[21]
- Cow's milk

The highest incidences of type 1 diabetes are found in northern Sardinia,

WHAT DO I DO IF MY BABY IS ALLERGIC TO MILK?

Cow's milk allergy is one of the most common in infants and young children, and is notorious for causing a wide variety of allergic symptoms. Identifying cow's milk allergy and removing milk from the diet of an allergic baby may appear easy enough, but deciding what to substitute for it is not. Currently, the two most commonly suggested substitutes are goat's or sheep's milk, and hydrolyzed (partially predigested and hypoallergenic) soy or milk protein formulas.

The challenge in all this is that infants allergic to cow's milk may be allergic to other foods and protein formulas, too. Consider this: allergic reactions to other foods, especially to soy, wheat, beef, peanuts, and citrus fruits develop in about 50 percent of proven cow's milk allergic infants.

Moreover, goat's or sheep's milk is not a good substitute for cow's milk in allergic babies. For example, one study of twenty-six young children with proven milk allergy found all the children were also allergic to goat's milk. Their immune systems couldn't distinguish the cow's milk protein, casein, from goat's or sheep's casein. In spite of this, some doctors continue to recommend goat's milk formulas for babies with cow's milk allergy.

When first commercially introduced, soy formulas were the only available substitute for cow's milk. Today, soy protein formulas are widely used alternatives for babies with proven cow's milk allergy, as well as high-risk allergy-prone infants when human breast milk is not available. However, you need to be aware that up to a third of all cow's milk allergic infants are also allergic to soy protein. You can find this out by giving your child an IgG food allergy test.

Without a doubt, breast milk is best. However, if breast-feeding is not an option, feeding with a hydrolyzed milk whey formula (milk protein with the highly allergenic milk protein casein removed) is associated with lower incidence of food allergies. There are also other low-allergenic milks available in health food stores, such as quinoa milk, rice milk, and almond milk, which are all reasonably high in protein, although they do not contain all the nutrients that specialized milk formulas are enriched with and therefore are not to be considered an alternative to breast milk or formula.

which fascinatingly has one of the world's highest rates of celiac disease (a severe form of gluten sensitivity), and in Finland, which is also the world's biggest consumer of dairy products.

Animal studies show that rats bred to be susceptible to diabetes have a much higher risk of getting the disease if their feed contains either milk or wheat gluten. In one study, even the addition of 1 percent skimmed milk to their diet increased the incidence of type 1 diabetes from 15 to 52 percent.

International research indicates that early and long-term avoidance of allergenic, "diabetogenic" foods, combined with a highly varied diet of wholesome and nonallergenic foods, can reduce a diabetic child's need for insulin by as much as two-thirds. So it's well worth having an IgG food allergy test to find out if you or your child are eating any offending foods.

Chapter 5

Food Allergy, Food Addiction, and Alcoholism

by James Braly, M.D.

"Sit down before Mother Nature as a small child. Be prepared
to cast aside all preconceived notions and to follow her
into whatever abyss she leads, or you shall learn nothing."

—*19th century biologist Thomas Huxley*

If you suffer from an IgG hidden food allergy, you are prone to food addiction; that is, you are likely to become addicted to those foods that are causing a delayed allergic reaction. Food allergy–induced food addictions in turn play a key role in a predisposition to and perpetuation of alcohol and drug abuse, chronic abstinence symptoms (long-term symptoms that often exist and persist when you're not drinking or using drugs), and a propensity to relapse into substance abuse over and over again.

When alcoholics stop drinking, their brain chemistry is still imbalanced and the cravings and other abstinence symptoms soon lead them elsewhere for a fix. Two substitutes commonly seen at AA meetings are pastries and coffee laced with sugar. Recovering alcoholics may also seek a high from binging and self-medicating on allergic-addictive foods, creating the same imbalanced and abnormal brain chemistry as the alcohol previously used (the opposite may also be true—recovering food addicts may turn to alcohol to help temporarily relieve the abstinence symptoms of food addiction).

In order to reduce your risk of abusing alcohol and drugs, and to become sober and remain sober, you must successfully address the problem of food allergy–food addiction as well.

IT ALL BEGAN WITH THERON RANDOLPH, M.D.

Theron Randolph, M.D., (1906–1995) was the founder of and leading pioneer in the field of environmental medicine and its subspecialty clinical ecology. He

47

is considered by many—myself included—as one of the outstanding allergists and clinicians of all time.

Dr. Randolph was the very first to propose that many physical and emotional symptoms and diseases are caused or aggravated by eating certain foods and exposure to environmental chemicals. He observed that food allergic people frequently develop physiological, maladaptive addictions to allergic foods, addictions associated with strong cravings. He observed that, at first, many food allergic people experience a pleasing addictive high, followed eventually by the development of tolerance, and acute withdrawal symptoms when they abruptly stop eating these same foods.

At the Fifth World Congress of Psychiatry in Mexico City in 1971, he stated:

[Allergic] foods eaten frequently and regularly are rarely ever suspected as [addictive] offenders. Persons addicted to common foods simply use them as often as necessary to keep well. In other words, "hooked" persons eat or drink their favorite "pick-me-ups" (food mixtures or primary foods) in order to remain "picked-up" (stimulated) and postpone or treat their "hangovers" (withdrawal effects). If food addictants are . . . eaten regularly, obesity, alcoholism, hyperactivity, insomnia, nervousness, and/or anxiety tend to develop; or persons may become self-centered, excited, aggressive, and agitated. . . . These developments, often called the "onset" of the present illness, usually prompt persons so affected to seek medical help.

I'd like to add depression to Dr. Randolph's list of conditions frequently seen in food allergic–food addicted individuals. For example, depression is one of the most common presenting symptoms in gluten sensitivity and celiac disease.

Dr. Randolph's findings were derived from over 20,000 patients interviewed and treated over a career spanning sixty years, and were expounded in his nearly 400 scientific articles.

DR. BRALY'S CLINICAL OBSERVATIONS, THEN AND NOW

During my clinical years in the 1980s, my staff and I would always begin with the assumption that patients entering our clinics with chronic medical conditions poorly responsive to conventional drug therapy were at high risk of having food allergies. Consequently, every patient was routinely tested for IgG food allergies. When we asked the patients to abruptly eliminate IgG allergic foods from their diets, about one-third experienced moderate-to-severe difficulty in getting through the first two or three days of abstinence. They universally complained of strong food cravings for the forbidden foods, and often reported a multiplicity of other symptoms as well, including but not limited to headaches, insomnia, irritability, depression, anxiety, shakiness, inability to concentrate, confusion, mental fogginess, and fatigue. If they gave in to their cravings and returned to the forbidden allergic foods—and, of course, some did—the symptoms abated immediately, not unlike an abstaining cigarette smoker or alcoholic giving in to the cravings.

Admittedly, at first, I found this concept difficult to accept, but as I observed it over and over again, it became undeniable that Dr. Randolph was right—many food allergic patients become addicted to commonly eaten foods in their diets, and at the same time these foods are the underlying causes or aggravating factors in many of their chronic symptoms and diseases. When asked to go "cold turkey" off IgG food allergens, many addicted patients experience signs and symptoms of withdrawal, not unlike those I'm observing twenty years later in the alcohol and chemically dependent clients here at Bridging the Gaps treatment center in Winchester, Virginia (see Resources).

DISORDERS THAT ALCOHOLISM AND FOOD ALLERGY SHARE IN COMMON

Another fascinating piece to the addiction puzzle is that alcoholics and food allergic patients suffer from many of the same medical conditions. This suggests that alcoholism and food allergy may share common causes, common triggers, and/or common biochemistry and physiology.

Let's look at a few of the more common of these shared disorders.

Attention Deficit Hyperactivity Disorder (ADHD)

In Chapter 4 we discussed the relationship between attention deficit hyperactivity disorder and IgG food allergies. IgG food allergy plays a key role in up to 80 percent of ADHD patients. Food allergy–induced ADHD is associated with a multiplicity of other, seemingly unrelated symptoms, such as food cravings, mood problems, conduct disorders, seizures, and digestive problems. Interestingly, when dealing with recovering alcoholics, one observes some of the same symptoms: food cravings, mood problems, seizures, and digestive problems.

In fact, ADHD occurs in the majority of alcoholics, according to Dr. David Miller and Merlene Miller, a husband-and-wife team with over twenty-five years of experience in the field of addictions, ADHD, and relapse prevention. In his pathbreaking book *Overload: Attention Deficit Disorder and the Addictive Brain* (Andrews and McMeel, 1996), Dr. Miller notes, "Significantly more children with attention deficit hyperactivity disorder (ADHD) develop problems with alcoholism or drug addiction than do children without ADHD. Alcoholics frequently have a history of childhood hyperactivity. People who become alcoholics show a much higher frequency of symptoms of ADHD as children than those who do not become alcoholics. Many people with ADHD are children of alcoholics and ADHD is common in the relatives of ADHD children. . . . It seemed reasonable to believe that, in many cases, ADHD and addiction were connected genetically."

I would add that if it's true that IgG delayed food allergies are a primary cause of ADHD in children and adults, then it seems reasonable to believe that ADHD, food allergy-food addiction, and alcoholism are connected genetically and biochemically. To treat alcoholism successfully, one must treat food allergy-food addiction successfully.

Shared Abnormal Brain Chemistry

One biochemical explanation for the occurrence of ADHD both among alcoholics and food allergy-food addiction sufferers is that both alcohol and food allergens are known to suppress the production and/or release of serotonin and dopamine. These two brain chemicals are thought to play a key role in the impulsivity, hyperactivity, and lack of concentration that are diagnostic of ADHD and commonly seen in recovering alcoholics.

Leaky Gut

As part of effective therapy in food allergic people, my staff and I would always insist that during "recovery" from food allergy-food addiction, no alcohol of any kind should pass the lips of patients. We instructed them that alcohol would prevent healing, prolong allergic reactions to foods, and result in failure of therapy.

The reason for this is that alcohol causes and aggravates a "leaky gut" (abnormal permeability or leakiness of the small bowel lining), and IgG food allergy, many experts agree, is triggered by a leaky gut. The problem is compounded by malnutrition and nutrient deficiencies that develop because of damage to the intestinal lining and suppressed digestion.

Depression

Depression that is unresponsive to antidepressant prescription drugs is a common presenting symptom of hidden food allergy (about 20 to 30 percent of depressed patients do not respond to prescription antidepressants; another 20 percent or so stop taking medications due to intolerable side effects). Some authorities claim that clinical depression is *the* most common presenting symptom in untreated celiac disease (remember that only about one in every thirty-nine Americans with celiac disease are diagnosed today).

Depression is also a common symptom in alcoholics, both while drinking and during sobriety. At Bridging the Gaps, we prefer taking clients off prescription antidepressants for at least thirty days after admission to see if the alcohol is causing the depression. Sometimes the depression vanishes simply because the recovering alcoholic remains sober. Other times, the depression persists even during long-term sobriety. Recovering addicts with persistent depression are at high risk of relapse.

Shared Abnormal Brain Chemistry

In general, low brain levels of serotonin and/or norepinephrine are the most common identified biochemical causes of depression. Low brain levels of these chemicals are found in food allergic, depressed patients and in recovering alcoholics. Simply eliminating food allergens such as gluten from the diet results in restoration of normal brain chemistry and may result in relief of depression in chronically depressed recovering alcoholics.

Insomnia and Snoring

Recovering alcoholics often complain of insomnia and many snore loudly. (Incidentally, the loudest snore ever recorded is well over 80 decibels, on par with the noise of a jackhammer!) People in recovery who struggle with sleep disorders and those who snore do not sleep deeply—that is, do not reach the restorative, healing, antiaging, growth hormone–releasing stage 4 sleep—and are at increased risk of relapse.

Food allergic–food addicted patients suffer from insomnia and snoring as well. Often the simple elimination of IgG food allergens allows an insomniac and recovering alcoholic to sleep soundly through the night and without snoring. Not incidentally, the same observation has been made with insomniacs and snorers who go on a three-day water or vegetable juice fast—in other words, a food-allergy-free diet.

Shared Abnormal Brain Chemistry

Recall that both food allergic–food addicted individuals and alcoholics share common abnormal brain chemistry. One of the brain neurotransmitters, serotonin, derived from the essential amino acid tryptophan and vitamin B_6, is naturally converted in the brain into the sleep hormone called melatonin.

Both food allergic–food addicted individuals and alcoholics suffer from differing degrees of malnutrition, including folic acid and other B-vitamin deficiencies. When you are B-vitamin deficient, both serotonin and melatonin production is badly compromised and sleep suffers.

Liver Damage

Alcohol damages the liver. Cessation of drinking allows the liver to heal in most cases. Heavy drinking severely injures the liver, leading to cirrhosis and eventually to liver failure.

Gluten-sensitive individuals also show evidence of liver injury (often labeled as "abnormal liver enzyme elevation of unknown cause") that is reversed simply by eating a gluten-free diet.

Shared Malnutrition

As a result of poor food choices, damage to the intestinal lining, a leaky gut, poor digestion, poor absorption of nutrients, and substituting alcohol for nutrient-dense calories, all alcoholics in early recovery are badly malnourished. As a result, natural body chemicals that protect the liver (hepatoprotective) and that help regenerated liver cells (hepatoregenerative) become deficient. Two such natural chemicals are SAMe (S-adenosyl methionine) and glutathione, both notoriously low in recovering alcoholics. Consequently, the liver becomes vulnerable to damage, scarring, and failure.

Allergic reactions to foods are associated with damage to the intestinal lining, a leaky gut, poor digestion, and poor absorption of nutrients. Food allergic–food addicted patients are malnourished (celiacs extremely so), and both SAMe and glutathione are reduced. Consequently, the liver becomes vulnerable to damage and has a reduced ability to heal.

21ST CENTURY THERAPY FOR ALCOHOLISM AND FOOD ADDICTIONS

Examining the similarities between food allergy–food addiction and alcoholism provides valuable insights that can help in the treatment of both of these conditions.

Intravenous and Oral Nutrient Therapy

Both food allergic–food addicted patients and recovering alcoholics have similar positive responses to intravenous (IV) and oral nutrient therapy.

In my previous clinic practice, when food allergic–addicted patients experienced strong withdrawal symptoms from forbidden foods, and were unable to continue with the food-elimination program, we often would place them on intravenous nutrient therapy (composed of high doses of vitamin C, B vitamins, magnesium, and calcium, administered or dripped in over one to two hours). The results were often extraordinary: unbearable withdrawal symptoms from allergic–addictive foods were dramatically reduced following the first or second IV drip.

Recovering alcoholics respond well to similar treatment. Six to ten days of nutrient therapy with high doses of intravenous vitamin C, activated B vitamins, magnesium, calcium, trace minerals, glutathione, the methyl donors methyl folate and dimethylglycine, and amino acid precursors is highly effective in quickly reversing and ameliorating the chronic abstinence symptoms common in recovering alcoholics (these include alcohol craving, sugar craving, salt craving, depression, anxiety, restlessness, fatigue, irritability, and brain fogginess). Refer to the "Abstinence Symptom Severity Scale" in Appendix 3 for a more complete list of chronic abstinence symptoms.

Dr. David Miller and I created the "Abstinence Symptom Severity Scale" for recovering alcoholics and chemically dependant clients. Most people in recovery have lingering, long-term symptoms of abstinence. The purpose of this scale is to measure and regularly monitor these symptoms semi-quantitatively. It is an invaluable tool to help the people in recovery and their therapists determine success or failure of therapy, and quickly signal impending danger or risk of relapse. Any symptom with a severity of 5 or above on the scale is considered noteworthy, 8 or above requiring immediate attention. A total score above 100 indicates a need for immediate intervention. Before IV/oral nutrient therapy total scores above 100 are common among recovering alcoholics and drug addicts. After one week of IV/oral therapy, most clients achieve and maintain total scores under 35, some under 10. (We are beginning to use this same scale to monitor food allergic–food addicted clients as well.)

The Wave of the Future Is Now

Conventional "talk" therapy for alcoholism is associated with a relapse rate (failure rate) of 75 percent or more within six months of therapy, and is no longer acceptable. Those of us making use of science-based alternative therapies for alcoholism are increasingly confident we have found an answer in the causal link between alcoholism, food allergy, and chemical imbalances in the brain: through nutritional therapy, we can address these three interrelated problems and aid brain cell repair. We no longer have to wait for the future to appear with dramatic breakthroughs. The future is now.

A number of years ago, Dr. Joan Mathews Larson introduced applied nutrition into her therapy for recovering alcoholics (see Dr. Larson's best-selling book *Seven Weeks to Sobriety,* published by Ballantine in 1992). By focusing on nutrition, Dr. Larson saw immediate improvement in outcomes: the relapse-free success rate skyrocketed from the shamefully low national average of 25 percent to a stunning 74 percent over a three-year period.

One of the key components of her revolutionary therapy was routine laboratory testing for IgG food allergies. What are the most common food allergens showing up in recovering alcoholics? You guessed it—wheat and dairy. According to Dr. Larson, once allergic-addictive foods are removed from the diet, "withdrawal symptoms [appear] as your body pleads for its usual fix of these foods. Symptoms vary from person to person and can include headache or fatigue during the first days. Back and joint aches may develop on the third day and persist for a day or two. Among the 'psychological' symptoms of [food allergy–food addiction] withdrawal are anxiety, confusion, depression, and mood swings. By the end of the week, withdrawal agonies, if any, will have ceased."

As more and more addiction centers, addictionologists, and counselors become familiar with and embrace the extraordinary value of IgG food allergy testing, rebalancing brain chemistry, and brain cell repair through nutrition, the sooner we will see relapse rates plummet and long-term sobriety become the rule rather than the exception.

KICKING THE FOOD ADDICTION–ALCOHOLIC HABIT

While struggling mightily with the symptoms of abstinence early in his career, professional golfer and recovering alcoholic John Daly was quoted as saying something to this effect: if how he felt while abstaining from alcohol was what sobriety was all about, he'd rather be drunk. If only the John Dalys of the world and their counselors would explore "the abyss" of food allergy–food addiction.

To reiterate, food allergy–food addiction and alcohol addiction share similar biochemical, maladaptive processes, resulting in similar and at times identical symptoms, diseases, and outcomes. This biochemical similarity explains why so many sober alcoholics continue to suffer the physical, mental, and emotional torment they expected to vanish into thin air when they stopped drinking. They are sober, but punished daily by the well-named, well-known beast called "white knuckling."

Identifying and eliminating hidden IgG allergic foods is only half the battle. Like an alcoholic drawn to binging and boozing and denial, you will still find these addictive foods appealing, in exactly the same way and for the same biochemical reason alcohol is appealing: they both promise a neurochemical high and/or relief from withdrawal symptoms. If you're beginning to see the similarity between this and the effects you or a loved one may be getting from alcohol, coffee, and/or cigarettes, you are finally beginning to understand the universal problem of food allergy–food addiction.

By being tested for IgG food allergies and kicking all of these hidden food addictions, you can put an end to the physical, mental, and emotional turmoil, the cravings, depression, and anxiety that entice you back for just one more quick fix—and then another fix—and if you're in alcohol recovery, make abstinence from alcohol much less painful and much more successful.

Chapter 6

The Top 20 Common Food Allergens

You are unique. That means that what you may or may not be allergic to is individual to you. That being said, after two decades and tens of thousands of IgG allergy tests, it's been found that certain foods are more likely to initiate allergic reactions than others. This does not necessarily mean that the food in question is "bad"—just that it's bad for you if you react. As you'll see in the next chapter, just about anybody can develop allergies to the foods they eat most often if the lining of the small intestine (that tennis-court-size layer of membranes inside you) has become much more permeable, or "leaky," allowing undigested food proteins to enter the bloodstream. Alcohol, aspirin, and aspirin substitutes (NSAIDs), overuse of antibiotics, prolonged stress of any kind, and gut infections or inflammations are common causes of gut leakiness.

Also, as we've seen, it is mostly proteins within food that the body's immune system reacts to. For example, some people react to fish or soy but not to fish oil or soybean oil. Others react badly to milk but not to butter. Those with dairy allergies often react worst to nonfat or low-fat milk, which has a higher relative protein content than whole milk, in which the fat actually slows down the absorption of the protein.

The twenty most common food or food group allergens are shown in the inset on the following page, in descending order. Of all these foods, by far the most common allergy-provoking substances are dairy products, yeast, eggs, and grains, especially wheat.

In the sections that follow, we'll explain why it may be unwise for anyone to eat three of the most common allergy-provoking foods—milk, wheat, and yeast—on a daily basis. And we'll explain what it is about other common foods that make them more likely than others to provoke allergy in some of us.

MILK—A FOUR-LETTER WORD?

Whichever way you look at it, cow's milk is consistently the most common food allergen. Classic IgE-based milk allergy is the most common food allergy, and so, too, is hidden or delayed-onset IgG milk allergy. A myriad of studies have shown that milk-sensitive people have much higher levels of IgG anti-

---

THE TOP 20 COMMON DELAYED-ONSET IgG FOOD ALLERGIES

1. Cow's milk—especially nonfat and low-fat milk

2. Gluten grains—found in wheat, rye, barley, oats, Kamut, spelt, and triticale

3. Gluten (gliadin)—found in wheat, rye, and barley, but not oats

4. Yeast—both baker's and brewer's yeast

5. Egg whites—children are most affected

6. Cashew nuts

7. Egg yolk—older adults are most affected

8. Garlic

9. Soybeans—prevalence of soy allergy is increasing by leaps and bounds

10. Brazil nuts

11. Almonds

12. Corn

13. Hazelnuts

14. Oats (contains gliadin-free gluten)

15. Lentils

16. Kiwifruit

17. Chili peppers

18. Sesame seeds

19. Sunflower seeds

20. Peanuts—be careful with this allergy, which is usually always fixed, permanent, and dangerous, even when small amounts are eaten

bodies that target milk proteins than people who are not sensitive to milk.[1-9] (As with gluten sensitivity and celiac disease, most people with high levels of IgG milk antibodies may be symptom-free early on, but often develop disabling symptoms later.)

Most cheeses, cream, yogurt, and butter contain milk protein, and it's hidden in all sorts of food. If you check labels, you'll find it's sometimes called simply milk protein, sometimes whey (which is milk protein with the casein removed), and sometimes casein or caseinate, which is the predominant type of protein—and the most allergenic—in dairy products. You'll be amazed at how many foods contain milk and casein—from bread and cereals to packaged food and chips. So if you're tested and find you're allergic to milk, you will have to be vigilant with processed foods.

Milk's status as an allergen isn't surprising. This is a highly specific food, containing all sorts of hormones designed for the first few months of a calf's life. It's also a relatively recent addition to the human diet. Approximately 75 percent of people (25 percent of people of Caucasian origin and 80 percent of Asian, Native American, or African origin) stop producing lactase, the enzyme that's needed to digest the milk sugar lactose, once they've been weaned—one of many clues that human beings aren't meant to drink cow's milk, at least beyond early childhood.[10] Lactase deficiency or lactose intolerance leads to diarrhea, bloating, cramping, and excess gas.

However, it's not the lactose that causes the allergic reaction. It's the protein. In other words, you can be either lactose intolerant, or milk-protein allergic, or both; and in fact, lactose intolerance and milk allergy often occur together.

Of course, most of us have been brainwashed by milk marketers since childhood into believing that milk is practically a wonder food. This can only leave you speculating how half the world, for example most of China and Africa, can survive, let alone thrive, without it. Milk is a reasonably good source of calcium, among other nutrients, but drinking milk certainly isn't the only way, or necessarily the best way, to achieve optimum nutrition. On top of that, it contributes to a wide range of common diseases.

Cow's milk is a major contributing factor to middle-ear infections (otitis media—see also page 41), an allergic disease that affects over a million of our babies and children each year. Milk allergy also contributes to iron deficiency, the most common nutritional deficiency in the world, by impeding the absorption of iron, and damaging the inside lining of the intestines, which causes slow blood leakage and a further loss of iron in red blood cells. In a quarter of people with iron deficiency, anemia can set in—seen in about 10 percent of children overall, 30 percent of children in inner cities, and as many as half of all children in poor countries.

Cow's milk is also one of the top two or three food allergens found in children and adults with poor sleep, asthma, eczema, migraines, rheumatoid arthritis, hyperactivity, bronchitis, more frequent infections, and longer hospital stays for premature infants, nonseasonal allergic rhinitis, bed-wetting, so-called growing pains, colic, heartburn, indigestion, chronic diarrhea, chronic fatigue, hyperactivity, depression, autism, epilepsy (although only in those with concomitant migraines and/or hyperactivity), and perhaps, as we saw in Chapter 4, even type 1 diabetes. The two most common food allergens in recovering alcoholics are milk and gluten grains, which may play a causative role in the disease (see Chapter 5). If you have ever suffered from any of the conditions mentioned above, milk should be high on your suspect list for a hidden food allergy. Iain's story bears this out.

CASE STUDY: IAIN

Seven-year-old Iain had suffered from chronic insomnia, extreme hyperactivity, and asthma all his life. His behavior was affecting his learning at school. An IgG food allergy test identified that he was allergic to milk. Iain had been in the habit of regularly drinking up to two pints of milk a day.

Within a week of cutting all dairy products from his diet, Iain's mother began to notice a difference in his behavior. He was less excitable, more settled, and could concentrate better. Over the following months, other problems began to reduce significantly. He began sleeping through the night and no longer needed steroid medication for his asthma. On the odd occasion when some milk slips into his diet, some of his behavioral problems and the insomnia return with a vengeance—thankfully, says his mother, only temporarily.

If you are allergic to cow's milk, goat's or sheep's milk are not a viable alternative. They all contain casein—the most allergenic of milk proteins—and your immune system is unlikely to be able to distinguish one milk from the other.

Getting Enough Calcium without Milk

If you're allergic to milk, getting the right amount of calcium becomes an issue of particular concern. After all, it is a fact that milk is a good source of both calcium and vitamin D, both of which are needed by the body to build healthy bones. No one who has seen elderly women severely bent over from osteoporosis of the spine can take the issue of calcium loss in the bones lightly. Yet a 1997 study found no connection between teenage consumption of calcium from cow's milk and the risk of bone fractures later on as an adult.[11] Other studies have concluded that the more dairy products a woman consumes, the more likely she will suffer from osteoporotic bone fractures![12-15]

Not all studies have revealed such findings, but the evidence for milk helping to build strong bones is far from clear-cut. The linear idea that bones contain calcium, and milk contains calcium, so milk must be good for the bones, crumbles in the light of recent research published in the *British Medical Journal*. This study shows that supplementing calcium makes no real difference to the risk of osteoporosis.[16] The study gave more than 3,000 woman aged seventy and over, all of whom were deemed to be at high risk for osteoporosis, supplements of 1,000 milligrams (mg) of calcium and 800 international units (IU) of vitamin D, or nothing. After two years there was no difference in fracture rate between those supplementing calcium and vitamin D and those who weren't. Despite all this, both the United States and United Kingdom governments help fund dairy industry campaigns to get kids and teenagers drinking more milk!

The simple truth is that we've become overly obsessed by the role of calcium deficiency in osteoporosis—an attitude that has driven an obsession with drinking that highly allergenic substance, milk. There are plenty of other factors that contribute to poor bone formation, reduced bone density, and osteoporosis: high blood pressure; undetected celiac disease; a diet excessively high in animal protein, including dairy; high caffeine consumption; excessive alcohol; excessive salt and refined sugar; lack of weight-bearing exercise; advancing age; and diets low in nutrients such as vitamins C, D, and K, and/or minerals such as magnesium, manganese, copper, boron, and silicon, as well as calcium. Even a lack of onions in your diet may accelerate bone loss!

All these areas are worth looking at in your life. In the meantime, how can you get that calcium? Table 6.1, "Common Sources of Calcium: How They Compare," shows you sources other than dairy products. See how milk products compare to these foods. If you start your day with (nonallergic) cereal and soy or rice milk or any other non-cow's milk fortified with calcium, and a heaped tablespoon of ground seeds, you've already achieved 404 milligrams (mg) of calcium. Have a few almonds and a bean dish during the day, with some broccoli, and you're up to 800 mg of calcium. That's the equivalent of two and a half glasses of milk. The recommended dietary allowance (RDA) of

TABLE 6.1. COMMON SOURCES OF CALCIUM: HOW THEY COMPARE

Milk—250 milliliters (ml) = 315 milligrams (mg) calcium
Firm cheese—50 grams (g) = 350 mg calcium
Yogurt—175 ml = 275 mg calcium

FOOD	SERVING	CALCIUM (MG)	RATING
Almonds	125 mg (½ cup)	(200)	**
Baked beans	250 mg (1 cup)	(163)	**
Beet greens, cooked	125 mg (½ cup)	(87)	*
Bok choi, cooked	125 mg (½ cup)	84	*
Brazil nuts	125 mg (½ cup)	130	*
Bread, whole wheat or white	1 slice	25	
Broccoli, cooked	125 mg (½ cup)	38	
Cauliflower, cooked	125 mg (½ cup)	18	
Chickpeas, cooked	250 mg (1 cup)	84	*
Dates	60 mg (¼ cup)	12	
Figs, dried	4 medium	61	*
Kale, cooked	125 mg (½ cup)	103	*
Lentils, cooked	250 mg (1 cup)	40	
Nuts, mixed	125 mg (½ cup)	48	
Orange	1 medium	52	*
Prunes, dried, uncooked	60 mg (¼ cup)	18	
Raisins	60 mg (¼ cup)	21	
Red kidney beans, cooked	250 mg (1 cup)	(52)	*
Rhubarb, cooked	125 mg (½ cup)	(184)	**
Rice, white or brown	125 mg (½ cup)	12	
Rice drink (fortified)	250 mg (1 cup)	300	***
Salmon, canned with bones	½ 213 g can	225	**
Sardines, canned with bones	½ 213 g can	210	**
Sesame paste (tahini)	30 mg (2 tbsp)	(40)	
Sesame seeds	125 mg (½ cup)	(104)	*
Shrimps, cooked/canned	70 g (12 large)	41	
Soybeans, cooked	125 (½ cup)	(93)	*
Soy drink	250 mg (1 cup)	28	
Soy drink (fortified)	250 mg (1 cup)	300	***
Spinach, cooked	125 mg (½ cup)	(129)	*
Tofu, regular processed†	100 g (⅓ cup)	(150)	*
White beans, cooked	250 mg (1 cup)	(170)	**

( )—Calcium from these foods is known to be absorbed less efficiently by the body.

† The calcium content shown for tofu is an approximation based on products available on the market. Calcium content varies greatly from one brand to the other and can be quite low. Tofu processed with magnesium chloride also contains less calcium.

Rating as established according to Canadian Food and Drug Regulations:

* Source of calcium

** Good source of calcium

*** Excellent source of calcium

Source: Health Canada, Canadian Nutrient File, 1993

calcium for an adult is 800 mg, and most decent multivitamins will provide a further 200 mg. So, there's no need to go short if you eat a healthy diet free from dairy products, but you do need to know what to eat.

WHEAT, GLUTEN, AND GLIADIN— THE INFAMOUS CEREAL KILLERS?

Your daily bread may be your deadly bread, and you may not even know it. Wheat, some other grains and the cereal proteins gluten and gliadin could be a big factor in any feelings of unwellness you're experiencing.

Hidden Risk—Celiac Disease

The old view was that about 1 in 5,000 people had celiac disease, the genetically transferred digestive and malnutrition disorder caused by an extreme allergy to gluten. However, new research shows that gluten allergy affects possibly as many as 1 in 100 normal, symptom-free people, often showing no digestive symptoms at all, and as many as 1 in 10 people with type 1 diabetes, thyroid disease, Down's syndrome, and first-degree family members of a known celiac disease victim.

Go back ten years and celiac disease was diagnosed by gut biopsy to see if the villi—tiny finger-like protrusions in the intestine walls that aid nutrient absorption—had shrivelled up and flattened. Nowadays, it's most easily diagnosed by a simple blood test called the IgA anti-tissue transglutaminase test, or tTG for short. Other tests for celiacs are discussed in Chapter 7.

When this test for celiac disease was randomly carried out on school-children, undiagnosed and unsuspected celiac disease was found to occur in 1 in every 167 so-called normal, healthy children and 1 in every 111 normal, healthy adults.[17] Among those who report gastrointestinal symptoms, it occurs in 1 in 40 children and 1 in 30 adults. Among those who have a father, mother, brother, sister, or grandparent with celiac disease, the risk is 1 in 11. So the condition is far from rare. In fact it is a very common—and commonly undiagnosed—disease in the United States and Britain.

However, many more people are allergic to wheat and other gluten grains, but don't have and will never have celiac disease. This is often because their immune systems produce IgG antibodies that attack wheat, or a component of it, producing a whole host of insidious delayed symptoms that somehow never develop into full-blown celiac disease.

COMMON SYMPTOMS OF GLUTEN ALLERGY

- Chronic or recurring upper respiratory tract problems like sinusitis and "glue ear"
- Chronic fatigue caused by malabsorption of nutrients
- Chronic fatigue syndrome
- Mouth ulcers (canker sores)
- Anemia, including iron, folic acid, B_{12}, and B_6 deficiency anemia
- Osteoporosis (especially if poorly responsive to conventional therapies)
- Unintended weight loss
- Short stature in children
- Iron-deficiency anemia
- Chronic diarrhea
- Constipation
- Abdominal bloating
- Crohn's disease
- Diverticulitis
- Depression (especially if poorly responsive to antidepressant medications like Prozac, Zoloft, or Paxil)
- Attention and behavioral problems in children, including ADHD
- Autism

So what are the symptoms of gluten allergy? The inset on page 63 gives the most common ones. Remember, however, that many gluten-sensitive people have no digestive symptoms at all. If you have a number of these symptoms, or risk factors, we strongly advise you to get tested (see next chapter).

The Trouble with Wheat

Wheat is a big staple in our diets. Some 600 million tons of it are eaten every year, and as breads, bagels, pancakes, biscuits, pastas, and so on, it makes up about one-third to one-half the average person's diet. So the idea that it isn't good for you may be difficult to swallow. However, a look at our history tells a different story.

Species take a very long time to adapt to any new food. We humans have a genetic record stretching back 250,000 to one million years or more. Humans started eating gluten grains, at the earliest, 10,000 years ago. So if the history of mankind was condensed into twenty-four hours, we've been eating gluten grains for, at most, fifteen minutes. Some cultures only started eating wheat in the last 100 to 200 years—the last four seconds. Thanks to advances in DNA research, we now know that humans shrank in height and head circumference when they shifted to primarily a grain-eating diet. Our hunter-gatherer ancestors, living on meat, fish and seafood, vegetables, fruit, nuts, and seeds, were five to six inches taller than those early farmers, and had brains 11 percent bigger.

Recently, it has been discovered that people with gluten allergies have a genetic "tag" located on the surface of white blood cells. This tag is called DQ2 and DQ8, which is common in societies that introduced grains late—notably the northwest and far north of Europe, especially western Ireland, Iceland, Finland, and Scandinavia, where grain growing isn't easy. This research is revealing that as many as one in three people in Ireland, Wales, England, and Scotland may be allergic to gluten. The Finnish population appears to be even more allergic.

Knowing all this, you might wonder why we are eating so much wheat. The answer is simply that bakers the world over love to work with cereals that have a high gluten content (Canadian hard wheat is an international favorite for this reason). The higher the gluten content, the more elastic, malleable, expandable, and heat resistant the dough becomes. This results in lighter, softer, more visually attractive, delicious tasting, and profitable breads, bagels, pastas, biscuits, and pastries.

A worrying trend in the United States, where "low-carb" diets are a craze, is to remove the carbohydrates from wheat products so you're just eating the protein. As this is principally gluten, it's a recipe for disaster for anyone with a hidden gluten allergy. So popular have high-gluten products become in the modern diet that wheat products represent three of the top six foods, in terms of calories consumed, of both the British and Americans—the other three are dairy products. So, what's the alternative?

While gluten is the key protein in wheat, it's also found in rye, barley, and oats. In fact, gluten is a name for a family of proteins found in grains. The principal type of gluten in wheat is called gliadin, followed by glutenin,[18] while the main type of gluten in rye is called hirudin, and in barley, secalin, although both also contain some gliadin. These are similar chemically, so a person who is sensitive to wheat is more likely to react to rye than barley. The type of gluten found in oats, however, bears no resemblance to gliadin. Approximately 80 percent of people diagnosed with celiac disease don't react symptomatically to oats.[19-20]

If you suspect you might be gluten sensitive, you could start by avoiding all gluten grains (wheat, rye, barley, and oats) for at least one month. Remember, however, that gluten is hidden in some 2,000 different processed foods. If this avoidance diet makes you feel noticeably better, you could then try reintroducing oats, since oats contain no gliadin, and see what happens.

About one in three people tested using an IgG food intolerance test will react to wheat. Of these, 90 percent will react to gliadin, while 15 percent will react to barley and 2 percent to rye. Even fewer react to oats. We think it's well worth getting yourself checked out with an IgG blood test from a reliable, licensed laboratory. It saves a lot of guesswork.

Most people's immune systems, and that may mean you, react to gliadin when it gets into the bloodstream. After all, as we saw above, it's an alien protein that hasn't been around for long in human existence. Research shows that at least 15 percent of wheat eaters do have antibodies against gliadin in their blood. Of course, if you have good genes, don't eat wheat, rye, or barley very often, have impeccable digestion and a superhealthy digestive tract, gliadin will not enter your bloodstream and cause an allergic response.

In Table 6.2 on page 66, you can see which grains contain gluten and which do not. (Note that spelt, Kamut, and triticale are all forms or hybrids of wheat.)

Going Gluten-Free?

If you have any of the common symptoms of gluten allergy, and have proven IgG allergic to wheat gluten and gliadin, it's well worth getting tested for celiac disease (see Chapter 7). As Pat shows, it's never too late to test.

TABLE 6.2. GLUTEN AND NON-GLUTEN GRAINS	
GLUTEN GRAINS	**NON-GLUTEN GRAINS**
Wheat	Buckwheat
Spelt	Corn
Rye	Millet
Barley	Teff
Oats (no gliadin)	Rice
Kamut	Quinoa
Triticale	Amaranth

CASE STUDY: PAT

Pat suffered from unexplained chronic iron-deficiency anemia, weight loss, fatigue, lower back pain, premature osteoporosis, gastrointestinal bleeding, bloating, and loss of appetite. After thirty-five years of these debilitating symptoms, Pat was diagnosed with celiac disease—confirmed by both blood tests and biopsy. Within three months of excluding gluten from her diet, her iron levels normalized, her energy level returned to normal, she regained her appetite, and she achieved a normal body weight.

If, after testing, you prove to be in the 15 to 20 percent of people with gluten sensitivity, or are one of the 1 in 111 apparently healthy adults who actually have celiac disease, you'll need to give up all the gluten in your diet. If that sounds easy, prepare for a shock.

You will discover that gluten is found in literally thousands of processed, packaged foods. Just go to your local supermarket and start reading labels—there's wheat in soups, sauces, gravies, sausages, and hundreds of other unsuspected foods; "modified food starch," often another name for gluten-contaminated food, is also found everywhere. Soon you will realize just how much our modern food-production system relies on gluten, and what a challenge it is to make your diet truly gluten-free.

You will have to begin by avoiding all bread and pasta products, doughnuts, pies, and cakes. Biscuits, pancakes, waffles, pizza, bagels, muffins, rolls, and baked goods of any kind will have to go, unless clearly and credibly labeled "gluten-free." Eating in restaurants can also be very challenging. Your best bet is to eat simply—whole foods without sauces, coatings, or gravies, such as steamed vegetables, fresh fruits, a baked potato with butter, or simply prepared baked or grilled fish. Be sure to ask your waiter or the chef a lot of questions! It may sound tough, but it's vital: it takes less than half a gram of gluten a day to cause toxic inflammation and cell death in your intestines.

If you'd like to know more about celiac disease, see Appendix 4; or for an in-depth treatment of this condition and wheat allergy, read Dr. Braly's *Dangerous Grains* (coauthored by Ron Hoggan, Avery, 2002).

BAKER'S AND BREWER'S YEAST— PROBLEM ON THE RISE

Yeast, the source of the next most widespread food allergy, is found not only in bread as baker's yeast, but also in soy sauce, beer, and, to a lesser extent, wine. Beer and lager are fermented with brewer's yeast. If you've noticed that you feel worse after beer or wine than you do after spirits—the "cleanest" being vodka—then you may be yeast sensitive.

Does this mean you can't drink? Not at all, assuming you are not an alcoholic or in recovery: it just means you'll need to pick and choose. Stick to spirits, or have a glass of champagne—made by a double-fermentation process, there's much less yeast in it. It's a good idea to limit your consumption of alcohol overall, though. Alcohol irritates the digestive tract and damages the liver, making it more permeable and vulnerable to undigested food proteins. This increases your chances of developing an allergic reaction to most anything, and it's why some people feel at their worst when they eat foods they're allergic to *and* drink alcohol. For example, you might be mildly allergic to wheat and milk and feel fine after either. But when you have both (pasta with cream sauce, for example), plus alcohol, you don't feel great. This combination often will provoke excessive mucus, abdominal bloating, migraine headaches, or asthmatic attacks.

Some people think they are allergic to wheat because they feel worse after eating bread. If you've noticed this—perhaps feeling sluggish, tired, bloated, or blocked up—but feel fine after pasta, you may not be allergic to wheat, but to the yeast in bread. This is what happened to Janette.

CASE STUDY: JANETTE

Over seven years, Janette's weight shot up 42 pounds, from 147 to 189 pounds, even though she stuck strictly to a low-calorie diet and exercised regularly. Not only was she heavier than before, but she also felt constantly tired and uncomfortably bloated after meals, particularly when she'd eaten bread. An IgG food allergy test showed she was allergic to yeast, milk, corn, soy, and haricot and kidney beans—but not to wheat. Simply by avoiding these foods, and without counting calories, Janette lost 28 pounds in five months!

Getting tested, in short, is the only way to be sure.

NUTS AND BEANS—SEEDS OF DESTRUCTION?

Nuts and beans are part of the same food family, along with fruit pips (small hard seeds found in certain fruits such as apples, pears, and cherries). Essentially, they're all seeds. The most common individual allergens in this group are, in descending order: peanuts, soybeans, cashew nuts, Brazil nuts, almonds, and hazelnuts. You can react to one and not others, but if you do react to a member of this family there's a greater chance that you'll react to another. Coffee and chocolate, both of which originate as beans, are also members of this family.

The most common immediate-onset, IgE allergy-causing foods are peanuts and tree nuts (such as almonds, walnuts, pecans, and cashews), according to the United States–based Food Allergy and Anaphylaxis Network (FAAN). About 1.5 million people in the United States and a possible 300,000 in the United Kingdom are allergic to peanuts (not a true nut, but a legume—in the same family as beans, peas, and lentils). Half of those allergic to peanuts are also allergic to tree nuts, and often sunflower and sesame seeds. Research is also reporting that allergy to soy, a novel food for many Westerners, is rapidly increasing, approaching the incidence of peanut allergy in Europe and the United States.

Unlike allergies to other foods like milk and eggs, children generally don't outgrow allergies to peanuts or nuts. But over time, they should become experienced at avoiding the foods that make them ill.

Recognizing and Diagnosing a Nut Allergy

The first signs of an immediate allergic reaction can be a runny nose, a skin rash or hives all over the body, or a tingly tongue. The symptoms may quickly become more severe and include signs of anaphylaxis (a sudden, potentially severe allergic reaction involving various systems in the body), such as difficulty breathing, swelling of the throat or other parts of the body, a rapid drop in blood pressure, and dizziness or unconsciousness. Other possible symptoms include tightness of the throat, shortness of breath, coughing, a hoarse voice, nausea, vomiting, abdominal pain, diarrhea, and lightheadedness.

To a person with no allergies, seeing someone else experiencing anaphylaxis can be just as scary as it is for the allergic person. What's more, anaphylaxis can happen just seconds to a few minutes after exposure to the allergen. It can involve various areas of the body (the skin, respiratory tract, gastrointestinal tract and cardiovascular system), and can be mild to fatal. The annual incidence of anaphylactic reactions is small—about thirty per 100,000 people—although people with asthma, eczema, or hay fever are at greater risk of having them.

Obviously, babies can't tell their parents when their heads or tummies hurt or their throats itch, so diagnosing food allergies early in a child's life can be difficult. We therefore generally recommend that parents refrain from giving their children peanut butter or other peanut or nut products until after they're two years old. If there's a family history of food allergies, parents should wait until the child is three. And many doctors recommend that their pregnant patients—especially those with food allergies—keep the lid on the peanut butter jar until after the baby is born and they've finished breast-feeding. Whenever possible, babies should be exclusively breast-fed at least until the age of six months; this is recommended to prevent or delay the appearance of food allergies.

If your doctor suspects your child might have a peanut or nut allergy, he or she will probably refer you to an allergy specialist for further testing because, as we've seen, the reactions can be very dangerous, even fatal. The allergy specialist will ask you and your child questions, such as how often your child has the reaction, what kind of reaction he or she has, how severe the reaction is, how quickly symptoms start after eating a particular food, and whether any family members have allergies or conditions like eczema and asthma.

SOY—FRIEND OR FOE?

Soy is something of a byword for health these days. Soy protein, isoflavones (plant-based compounds found in soy products), soybean oil, and fiber have been found to reduce the risk of developing menopausal problems, breast and prostate cancer, and cardiovascular risk—probably by reducing "bad" LDL cholesterol, triglycerides (blood fats), and other culprits. As such, it could benefit many type 1 diabetics who are concerned about the high risk of coronary artery disease their condition carries.

This array of benefits has prompted most nutrition experts to jump on the soy bandwagon. And there's more. Along with all soy's remarkable disease-fighting attributes (at least in Asian subjects, that is), vegetarians claim that it's a healthy and "ethical" milk and meat substitute. So where's the problem?

As with any food, if you're allergic to it, it's bad news. And soy allergies and soy-induced illnesses are unfortunately very common. With soy consumption rapidly on the rise in the United States and Britain (tripling over the last three years as it appears in more and more processed foods, from hamburgers, sausages, and salad dressings to chicken nuggets and breakfast cereals), there is an escalating increase in reports of allergic reactions. The reason for the explosion in soy allergy isn't completely known, but one proposed explanation is that because soy was introduced to the United States and Britain relatively recently, many people in these countries are genetically prone to reject its novel proteins. Another intriguing explanation is that genetically modified (GM) soy is more likely to cause allergies, and GM soy use has risen sharply in recent years.

The adverse effects can be very serious. If babies allergic to soy are introduced to it early in life (perhaps as an alternative to formula milk if they weren't breast-fed), that can actually increase the risk of developing type 1 diabetes. Along with wheat and milk casein, soy is considered by some researchers to be a leading diabetes-causing food.

Like peanuts, soy can also induce anaphylaxis in people severely allergic to it. In fact, soy and peanuts often cross-react—that is, the immune system has trouble distinguishing one from the other, and an allergy to peanuts is associated with a disproportionate degree of soy allergy, and vice versa.

By the way, soy and other beans and lentils are high in a type of carbohydrate called glucosides. These are quite hard for most of us to digest, but not for the bacteria within our guts. The net result is that they produce gas and possible bloating. But this does not necessarily mean that you are allergic. First, try chewing them more thoroughly. There's nothing like inadequate chewing of beans and lentils for producing gas. You could also go to a health food store and buy a digestive enzyme containing amyloglucosidase (also called glucoamylase), which helps you digest beans. If this relieves the embarrassing symptoms, there's no reason to assume you are allergic, unless other allergic symptoms—which for soy can include sinusitis and rhinitis—remain.

If you aren't allergic, it's good to know that some soy products are easier to handle than others (the Far East is awash in soy, after all). Soybeans themselves contain a number of "anti-nutrients" that make them hard to digest and also impede the absorption of other nutrients. Enzyme inhibitors in the beans, for instance, get in the way of the body's digestion of protein and phytic acid, which results in reduced absorption and bioavailability of iron and zinc. Soy is also high in lectins, which can irritate the gut; it's likely, in fact, that soy allergy is really a soy lectin allergy. But some soy products are low in lectins: fermented soy foods such as miso, natto, or tempeh have a fraction of the amount. So, too, does tofu. Some brands of soy milk also have low levels of these substances.

If you are considering a soy-based diet, perhaps because you're a vegan or are allergic to milk, our advice is first to get tested with an IgG food allergy test.

EGGS—A SCRAMBLED TALE

Like soy, eggs are an excellent source of high-quality protein, vitamins, minerals, the carotenoid lutein (which may help prevent cataracts and macular degeneration in the elderly), and also contain other important nutrients such as choline, which is vital for the brain. Also like soy, eggs can provoke allergic reactions. These egg allergies are particularly common in children. In one study of 107 children with allergic dermatitis, 92 were found to be allergic to egg white.[21] Egg allergy is certainly worth suspecting if you have either eczema or dermatitis, and eliminating eggs from the diets of children prone to eczema has proven effective.[22]

In another study investigating 156 children with the symptom of swollen lips, half were found to be allergic to egg white.[23] Egg white allergy is common, causing both immediate-onset IgE-mediated reactions (wheezing, skin rashes, and so on) as well as delayed IgG reactions. Reactions to egg white are much more common than to egg yolk, almost certainly because of a type of protein in egg white called ovomucoid. When ovomucoid is experimentally removed from egg white, most egg-allergic people stop reacting.[24] Eggs also contain certain enzyme inhibitors.[25]

It is possible that egg allergy is more common because egg, like milk, is very often introduced prematurely into infants' diets. Egg allergy is less common in adults.

GARLIC, CHILI, AND KIWIFRUIT—PUNGENT PERIL

The health benefits of garlic have been known for centuries, but remember—we are each unique, and this pungent bulb doesn't suit everybody. If you do test allergic to garlic, also be suspicious of onions, since they come from the same food family and many share common protein allergens. Another common culinary allergen is chili and, as it's part of the same family as cayenne and paprika, be wary of these if you find you're allergic. Of all the fruits, the most common allergens are kiwifruit and citrus fruit. Allergic reactions to kiwi are especially common in those people allergic to latex (77 percent of those with latex allergy are also allergic to kiwi) and to birch tree pollen. (But obviously, don't give up these delectable vitamin-rich fruits unless you've tested positive for them in an allergy test!)

While garlic, chili, and kiwifruit are among the most common foods to come up positive on an allergy test, it's important to recall that food allergies are unique to individuals. For example, in one trial testing 150 people with irritable bowel syndrome (IBS), only 23 people were found to be allergic to the same foods as another patient, but the remainder, that's 127 people, or 85 percent, had unique test results. In this trial, however, only one person failed to react to *any* of the top five allergenic foods.[26]

If this trial is anything to go by, it means that the chances you may be reacting to one of the top five foods are high—but also that the chances you react to *only* one of the top five are very small indeed. That's why we recommend you get yourself properly tested.

Chapter 7

◄◦►

Diagnosing
Your Food Allergy

As we explained in Chapter 2, there are two main kinds of food allergy: the immediate-onset, type 1, IgE antibody-based allergy, and the delayed-onset, type 3, IgG antibody-based allergy. Here's the lowdown on how to test for both.

IgE TESTING

Doctors use different kinds of tests to identify this rarer form of food allergy. When using skin testing, the doctor or nurse applies a dilute solution containing a food extract to the skin—often on the back or forearm. The skin is then scratched or punctured, allowing the food to penetrate the surface. If the person has an IgE allergy to that food, a positive reaction will take the form of a red bump resembling a mosquito bite, which appears in fifteen to twenty minutes.

There is also a blood test, popularly known as the IgE RAST (radioallergosorbent) test, which is of about the same diagnostic value as the skin test, and its spin-off, the IgE MAST test. They both measure serum levels of food-specific IgE antibodies. Skin tests and IgE RAST or MAST tests *only* detect IgE food allergies, not the more common IgG type.

In our opinion, the best test for IgE allergies is the IgE ELISA test. ELISA (enzyme-linked immunosorbent assay) is a laboratory technique also used for IgG food allergy testing. Exactly how it works is explained on page 77. The ELISA test is available from any allergy specialist, if you've been referred by your doctor, or from a number of laboratories listed in Resources. However, don't forget that IgE food allergies are far rarer than IgG food allergies, making this a less useful test unless you have severe and immediate reactions to food.

IgG TESTING

If you are chronically ill but have no firm diagnosis of the cause, if you find yourself going back again and again to your doctor without much long-term relief of symptoms, a vital first step on the road to optimum health is to suspect that a delayed-onset IgG food allergy may be involved. The crucial second step is to accurately identify and eliminate the relevant food allergens.

It should come as no surprise, however, that diagnosing delayed-onset food allergies has been fraught with seemingly insurmountable challenges. The symptoms of this kind of allergy show up gradually, in many forms and in many regions of the body, and can be triggered by a number of commonly eaten foods. The picture is muddied further because eating the allergen can actually make you feel better temporarily—a phenomenon sometimes known as food allergy–food addiction (discussed in Chapter 5)—and may not even provoke an allergic reaction every time you eat it. The sufferers' tales of woe about visits to one doctor after another are commonplace. Here are a couple of classic quotes we've often heard:

> "I was skin tested for food allergy and nothing showed up allergic, only to be told later that skin tests were inaccurate tests for most food allergies."
>
> "Once I was tested and found I was allergic to oranges, but not to wheat. The next month I took another test that said I was allergic to wheat but not to oranges. That's when I gave up."

How IgG Testing Evolved

For decades, the focus in this field was on "true" food allergies—namely, the IgE immediate-onset kind—and the diagnostic tool of choice was the skin test. But skin testing and IgE RAST blood testing don't work when it comes to detecting IgG food allergies.

It wasn't until the 1980s that published research began to demonstrate that a fundamental mechanism behind IgG food allergy was the penetration of large molecules of incompletely digested food through a leaky intestinal lining into the bloodstream. As food allergens enter the bloodstream, we were being told, IgG antibodies, not IgE, were forming against them.

As we saw in Chapter 2, IgG antibodies bind to the allergens, forming food allergen-antibody immune complexes. These immune complexes circulate throughout the body, and if not gobbled up by the detoxifying immune cells called macrophages, they will penetrate the walls of small blood vessels in various vulnerable sites in the body. Once firmly entrenched, immune complexes become sources of constant irritation, inflammation, and, ultimately, dysfunction and destruction of body tissues. Diseases such as food allergy-induced rheumatoid arthritis can then develop.

Since the gut lining never functions perfectly as a barrier at the best of times, the big difference between a food allergy sufferer and a nonallergic person appears to be the amount of partially digested food that reaches their bloodstream, and how well their immune system clears these allergens from circulation. If a lot of these foods get in over time, and kick-start the formation of many immune complexes, the person will inevitably begin to suffer from an IgG food allergy.

In the IgG test, a sample of blood is drawn and tested for the presence of IgG antibodies formed against foods in your diet. You can have your blood drawn at the offices of doctors familiar with IgG food allergy and blood tests or you can obtain home test kits like the one shown in Figure 7.1 from health clinics and some doctors. They contain a simple, almost painless device to obtain the pinprick of blood.

If you choose to do your own IgG ELISA test at home, you might want to get someone else to get the blood sample; although it doesn't hurt, it can be

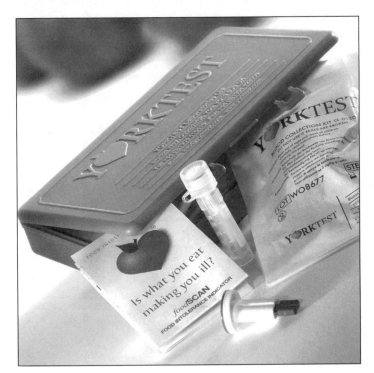

Figure 7.1.
Home test kit,
blood collection.

easier if you avert your eyes! Ask them to prick your finger on the side, which has fewer nerve endings than the pad. You then carefully place a tiny column of absorbent material against the drop of blood. You send this off to the laboratory by first-class or registered post, and provided it gets there within seventy-two hours (three days), it's accurate.

Warning: Not all laboratories are created equal. If you go through a doctor's clinic for the IgG blood test, ask the doctor if he periodically does "split sampling" to assure lab quality control. Split sampling is when the doctor draws two tubes of blood from the same patient, but unbeknownst to the lab sends the samples to the lab under two different names. The two samples should come back with similar results. If the doctor does not regularly send in split samples, the reliability of the test results are always suspect.

Depending on the lab, they can test the blood sample simultaneously against 100 or more foods. The blood is then exposed to tiny containers or wells, each containing a different food protein (see Figure 7.2 below).

In Figure 7.2 you can see which food proteins have caused a reaction, some more than others. If your blood serum contains abnormally high levels of IgG antibody against a particular food, it means you are allergic to that food. When this happens, as we've seen, the antibody and protein form a complex. The more complexes, the greater the density of the solution becomes. A light is then shone through the containers and the test results are read and recorded by computerized laboratory equipment.

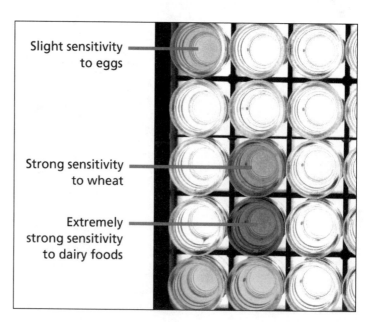

Figure 7.2. Petri dish panel marked up.

Slight sensitivity to eggs

Strong sensitivity to wheat

Extremely strong sensitivity to dairy foods

The IgG ELISA test measures degrees of reaction, which are graded from +1 to +4, with +4 being the strongest reaction. So when you get your result, you know exactly what you react to and the strength of your reaction. As this is a quantitative measurement, this kind of testing is called quantitative IgG ELISA food allergy testing. You should accept no other.

A sample report is shown in Figure 7.3. For example, if you have a +3 reaction, you need to avoid the food completely. If, on the other hand, you have only a marginal reaction, you will be advised to rotate that food—that is, eat it

foodSCAN 113 in-depth test : 05/12345 EXAMPLE2   **Y♥RK**TEST

Client Name : Mr Example Results

Test Date : Friday, 26 August 2005

	AVOID	ROTATE	NO REACTION
Grains	Wheat +2		Barley Buckwheat Corn (Maize) Gluten (Gliadin) Millet Oat Rice Rye
Dairy	Cows Milk +3 Egg White +1		Egg Yolk
Meats			Beef Chicken Duck Lamb Pork Turkey
Fish			Crustacean Mix Mollusc Mix Oily Fish Mix Plaice / Sole Salmon / Trout Tuna White Fish Mix
Vegetables			Asparagus Aubergine Avocado Carrot Celery Cucumber Haricot Bean Kidney Bean Lentils Lettuce Mushroom Mustard Mix Onion Pea Peppers (Capsicum) / Paprika Potato Soya Bean Spinach String Bean
Nuts		Almond Brazil Cashew	Coconut Hazelnut Peanut Walnut

Figure 7.3. Printout of an example of an allergy test result.

no more than every fourth day. In the next chapter we explain how to decrease your allergic tendency and reverse allergies, since you can grow out of most IgG food allergies if you know how.

The IgG ELISA test has many advantages:

- You don't have to fast overnight before taking the blood sample.

- It is relatively painless, involving just one skin prick.

- Over 100 different foods can be tested at the same time.

- It is largely an automated test, so if performed with the appropriate lab quality controls, it is accurate and reproducible.

The IgG ELISA test represents a step forward in the field of food allergy testing. It addresses the enormously prevalent problem of delayed food allergy head-on, and removes the barriers of inaccuracy and poor reproducibility that continue to plague many competing tests. It is our test of choice for diagnosing delayed-onset food allergies.

Consider the case of Patrick Webster, otherwise known as Mr. Sneezy because he holds the world record for sneezing in the *Guinness Book of World Records*. The IgG ELISA test turned his life around completely.

CASE STUDY: PATRICK WEBSTER

Patrick Webster's sneezing (nonseasonal allergic rhinitis) began when he was seventeen years old, and for the next thirty-five years of his life averaged roughly one sneeze every two minutes—that's 600 to 700 sneezes per day or 220,000 sneezes a year, amounting to about 7 million sneezes. So in the end, he had sneezed without interruption for 12,775 days! His relentless sneezing led to fatigue from lack of sleep, and forced him to retire early. Steroid therapy prescribed by his doctors has given him osteoporosis.

Webster finally heard about IgG food allergy testing. His test results revealed that he was allergic to oats, almonds, hazelnuts, milk, cheese, egg yolk, and tomatoes. He was not only a big cheese and milk consumer, but in addition, every morning of his adult life, he prepared his own muesli consisting of—you guessed it—oats, almonds, Brazil nuts, and cow's milk! When he eliminated the muesli and other offending foods, his sneezing stopped almost immediately and has not returned. For the first time in thirty-five years, Patrick is totally free of sneezing and nasal congestion and sleeps restfully through the night.

SCREENING FOR AND DIAGNOSING CELIAC DISEASE

We first looked at celiac disease—a digestive disorder caused by extreme allergy to gluten—in Chapters 3 and 6. We conservatively estimate that 30 million Americans and 6 million people in Britain are allergic to gluten cereals—wheat, rye, barley, oats, and the hybrids and variants triticale, spelt, and Kamut. One in 110 American adults has already developed celiac disease (the percentage is much higher among those with thyroid disease, insulin-dependent diabetes, or Down's syndrome, and those with a family member with celiac disease). If you do prove IgG sensitive to grains and gluten or gliadin, we recommend you also get tested for celiac disease. (For more details on this disease see Appendix 4, which we recommend you read if you are allergic to wheat.)

Many doctors regard the small-bowel biopsy as the "gold standard" for the diagnosis of celiac disease. It is commonly an outpatient procedure performed by a specialist. A long tube is inserted through the mouth, esophagus, stomach, and finally into the small intestine, where several biopsies of mucosa lining are taken. A pathologist looking for the characteristic lesions of celiac disease studies this tissue under a microscope.

As you can see, this procedure is an expensive, uncomfortable, and inconvenient diagnostic tool. Many doctors and their patients are understandably reluctant to have it performed unless there is very good reason for doing so. This is a primary reason why celiac disease continues to be underdiagnosed.

This is where modern laboratory science comes into play. Several antibody blood tests are currently being used with great success to help distinguish people who are likely candidates for celiac disease from those who aren't. As a result, many fewer unnecessary biopsies are being performed—saving in both costs and patients' suffering.

Since gliadin—the critical protein found in all gluten grains except for oats—appears to be the key offending protein to which celiacs react, testing to see whether a person is producing antibodies to gliadin can be used to screen for celiac disease. While we've been talking a lot about IgG antibodies, there's another kind of antibody, called IgA; and often people with celiac disease produce anti-gliadin IgA antibodies as well as anti-gliadin IgG antibodies. When you have an IgG food allergy test, one of the 100 or so potential food allergens you'll be tested for will be gliadin, so you'll have this information already.

Both the IgG and IgA tests are used to screen for celiac disease. The tests are done together in order to maximize the sensitivity of the screening—that is, to ensure that if you have celiac disease, one or both of the tests will pick it up well over 90 percent of the time. However, there is a problem with these tests. Even if you don't have celiac disease, one of the tests may still come up positive. You may be gliadin allergic, but not have celiac disease. Clearly, another, more specific screening test needs to be done.

The answer to the dilemma, at least at the moment, is the IgA anti-endomysium test. It is a more expensive and sophisticated screening test for celiac disease. Due to its expense, it is usually performed after one or both of the less expensive anti-gliadin antibody tests come back positive. It's more accurate, and if you have celiac disease, it comes up positive for IgA antibodies nearly 100 percent of the time. If you don't have celiac disease, it will come back negative approximately 95 percent of time.

A new test may soon replace this one: the IgA anti-tissue transglutaminase test, or tTG, also known as the TGA ELISA. This measures anti-transglutaminase IgA antibodies in human serum. Like the anti-endomysium assay, it is brought into play when either or both of the IgG or IgA anti-gliadin antibody tests are positive. Studies published in Europe and the United States confirm that the TGA is equivalent in accuracy to the anti-endomysium test.[1] If positive, it is very likely that you have celiac disease, and without question a follow-up intestinal biopsy is indicated for final confirmation. Our prediction is that the TGA will soon replace the anti-endomysium assay and may even replace small-bowel biopsies. Ask your doctor to run the TGA or anti-endomysium tests if you suspect you have celiac disease.

Chapter 8

———◄○►———

Why Allergies Develop and How to Prevent or Reverse Them

By now, we hope you will have decided to have a proper food allergy test to find out whether you have IgG or possibly IgE food allergies. But you might be feeling mixed emotions about it: excitement, because you could be pinpointing the source of your chronic ill health—and anxiety, because you feel a sense of loss about giving up favorite foods.

The good news is that you can grow out of most food allergies. While celiac disease and IgE-based food allergies are almost always fixed and permanent for life, most food allergies only involve IgG antibodies, and your immune system can "unlearn" its IgG sensitivities. If you strictly avoid a food you are currently IgG sensitive to for three to four months, there will be no more IgG antibodies left tagged for that food and the immune cells producing food-specific IgG antibodies appear to lose interest in doing so over time. This means you won't react allergically to that food when it's reintroduced.

Why not? It's because immune cells that produce IgG antibodies don't pass their "memory" on to the next generation. They often forget. Also, there are things you can do right now to decrease your sensitivity to food allergens. The way to reverse your food allergies is best understood by seeing how you developed them in the first place.

HIGH-RISK EATING

Have you ever wondered whether the food you eat actually wants to be eaten? In many cases it appears that it doesn't. Most food plants try their best to protect themselves from predators—with spikes, thorns, and chemical toxins. The idea that everything in a food is "good" is far from the truth. Most foods contain numerous natural toxins as well as beneficial nutrients.

Even foods that are obviously designed to be eaten can have this characteristic. For example, many fruits rely on animals eating them, so their seed can be spread in a ready-made manure bed—and thus widen their territory. However, the fruit has to protect itself from unwanted scavengers such as bacteria, viruses, or fungi that will simply rot the seed. So some seeds are hard to crack and toxic, such as apricot kernels, which contain cyanide compounds. For protective reasons, wild food contains a massive and often selective chemical arsenal to ward off specific foes. We and food have been fighting for survival since the beginning of time.

Our survival technique does have a few holes in it, though. Omnivores like us have a high-risk/high-return strategy, as far as food is concerned. We try different foods and if we don't immediately get sick, then it's okay to eat it. But this shortsighted test has failed us, many times. Gluten grains and cow's milk are prime examples of this. Indeed, even today, the average Western diet kills many people in the long run—although most of us are foraging in supermarkets rather than fields and woods.

WHY FOOD ALLERGIES ARE ON THE RISE

Before we show you how best to reduce your allergic potential, it's important to understand why food allergies are on the increase. Over the past 20,000 years, people have changed very little—and genetically, not at all. The same, however, cannot be said of our diets.

Many of today's killer diseases, from diabetes to heart disease, have arisen because our unchanging genetic constitution has collided head-on with a profoundly radical change in diet. Take a close look at this comparison between what our ancestors were eating 20,000 years ago and today's diet:

STONE AGE DIET	TODAY'S DIET
0% of carbohydrates as cereal grains (dietary wheat, corn, and rice didn't exist)	75% of carbohydrate as grains (rice, corn, and wheat head the list)
Favorite drinks: mother's milk, water	Favorite drinks: soft drinks, coffee, tea, alcohol, and cow's milk (20% of calories are now consumed as liquids)
Great variety of fruits and vegetables eaten	8 to 10 foods make up 80% of daily calories (dairy, wheat, refined sugars, fried potatoes)

Today we are drinking more high-sugar, fizzy drinks than water! Times have clearly changed. Are we becoming more food allergic simply because we are eating the wrong foods? When you consider that cow's milk, grains, and yeast are all essentially "new" foods in our human diet, this simplistic idea makes sense. Eating a monotonous diet of high-risk allergy foods is certainly part of the reason why food allergies are on the increase.

Consider the top nine foods eaten in the United States, rated by the number of calories consumed annually, as reported by the U.S. Department of Agriculture:

1. Full-fat cow's milk

2. Two percent-fat cow's milk

3. Processed American cheese

4. White (wheat) bread

5. White (wheat) flour

6. Rolls (wheat)

7. Refined sugar, which accounts for 15 to 21 percent of all calories

8. Soft drinks/fruit juices

9. Beef

Notice the absence of fruits and vegetables in this list. Notice also that dairy and wheat (gluten) products make up the top six foods. Recall that allergies to cow's milk and wheat are two of the most commonly reported. By eating these foods day in and day out, it's clear why so many people suffer from chronic food allergies over an entire lifetime. But it doesn't completely explain the phenomenon of food allergy.

Let's take a look at some other known factors that increase your chances of developing allergy and, if solved, will reduce your allergic potential:

- Increased intestinal permeability (leaky gut)

- Poor digestion

- Dysbiosis (lack of healthy gut bacteria)

- Lack of nutrients from poor diet

- Not being breast-fed

- Excessively clean environments during infancy and early childhood

- Use of antacids or antibiotics

- Having a parent with allergies

- Nonsteroidal anti-inflammatory drugs (NSAIDs)

- Regularly drinking alcohol

- Cross-reactions between different foods and airborne allergens

THE TOP FOOD ALLERGY PROMOTERS

Now let's examine each of these factors in detail. We'll also look more closely at addiction to problem foods.

Have You Got Leaky Gut Syndrome?

An obvious place to start in unraveling the true cause of allergies is the digestive tract. After all, the lining of the gut is the first point of contact between foods and your immune system. Did you know that the intestinal lining alone is estimated to contain more immune cells and produce more antibodies than any other organ in the body? Hardly surprising, then, that the intestinal lining and its immune system is an absolutely crucial defense against food allergens, food toxins, and food-borne infections.

Normally, the inner lining of your small intestine serves as a highly selective barrier against your internal environment, preventing the entry of potentially harmful toxins, microbes, and incompletely digested foods from the gut into blood circulation in much the same way that a bouncer keeps the riff-raff out of an exclusive club—which just happens to be your body. At the same time, this lining selectively allows the passage of important vitamins, minerals, amino acids, essential fatty acids, and other nutrients. It permits properly digested food protein, carbohydrates, and fats to easily gain entry into the bloodstream.

The trouble starts when this lining becomes more permeable or "leaky." Food particles can then enter the blood, and the immune system is exposed to proteins not on the guest list, so to speak, triggering an allergic reaction. Recent research shows that people with food allergies—and the medical conditions caused by food allergies—do tend to have leaky gut walls.[1] This might explain why frequently eaten foods are more likely to cause a reaction.

There are many reasons why our modern-day diet might lead to leaky gut. Consumption of alcohol, the frequent use of painkillers (anti-inflammatory drugs such as aspirin and ibuprofen), antibiotic use, excessive physical or emotional stress of any kind, a deficiency in essential fatty acids, or a gastrointestinal infection or infestation (such as candidiasis) are all possible contributors to leaky gut syndrome. If any of these apply to you, they'll need to be corrected in order to reduce your sensitivity to foods.

Moreover, eating foods you're allergic to is another major contributor to a leaky gut. That's right: hidden food allergies encourage more food allergies. So if you're wheat allergic and don't know it—and most people don't—it's probably making your digestive tract more permeable by irritating this inner skin every time you eat wheat. As a consequence, you may develop other food allergies, too.

A lack of key nutrients such as glutamine, vitamin A, essential fats, or zinc can also prevent proper integrity of the gut wall. More on these later because increasing your intake of key nutrients such as these can decrease your allergic potential.

You Are What You Digest

Food allergens also tend to pass through the digestive tract incompletely digested. This is because the digestive tract's natural tendency is to try to fend off any substance it perceives as harmful or toxic. So it attaches antibodies to the allergen to try, often successfully, to eliminate the food before it can pass into the bloodstream. The food passes out in the stool partially digested at best—and with it go the nutrients. This is one reason why some people with IBS can get diarrhea from eating foods they are allergic to. The end result is always suboptimal nutrition. So it can be said that the first basic requirement of optimum nutrition is a diet free of food allergens.

Developing food allergies becomes even more likely in people who don't produce enough of the right digestive enzymes. You release a pint or two of saliva and a staggering nine quarts of digestive juices, hopefully rich with digestive enzymes, into your stomach and intestines every day. Much of this fluid is reabsorbed. But if you lack sufficient enzymes, large amounts of big, undigested food molecules are reaching the gut wall. One research study of people with a sensitivity to man-made chemicals showed that 90 percent of them produced inadequate amounts of digestive enzymes, compared with 20 percent of healthy controls. If you regularly drink alcohol or are under constant stress, you also underproduce digestive enzymes, and as a consequence underdigest your foods.

Later on we'll tell you how supplementing digestive enzymes can have amazing effects on reducing your allergic potential. Zinc supplementation can also be helpful, as a deficiency in this mineral is extremely common among allergy sufferers. Zinc is not only needed for protein digestion, but is also essential for the production of hydrochloric acid in the stomach—and without enough stomach acid, you can't digest anything.

Beneficial Bacteria—The Inside Story

Inside the intestines there is a carefully balanced world of "friendly" and potentially "unfriendly" bacteria. The 180 friendly, health-promoting strains of bacteria are called probiotics. At last count they include a minimum of nine strains of *Bifidobacteria* and sixty-four of *Lactobacillus* bacteria.

Probiotic bacteria have many scientifically proven benefits, including:

- Preventing and treating food allergy

- Alleviating intestinal inflammation

- Preventing abnormal gut leakiness or permeability

- Preventing and reversing diarrhea caused by antibiotics, food allergy, and infections

- Suppressing IgE antibody production

- Protecting against or reducing the number of food allergy-provoking candida yeast infections (candidiasis)[2]

Much depends on that balance of probiotics with "bad" bacteria in the gut, however. If you were introduced to the wrong foods too early in life, or had a poor diet as a child or adult, perhaps with too high a sugar intake or alcohol consumption, or have overused antibiotics and other prescription drugs, it's easy to become deficient in probiotic bacteria, leaving room for disease-causing microbes to take over and dominate. As a result, your digestive tract may become prone to inflammation, leaving your gut leakier and impairing digestion.

Probiotic supplements can help to reverse this imbalance.[3] For example, a Finnish study found breast-fed infants with eczema and cow's milk allergy improved significantly when their mothers were given probiotic bacteria supplements. The report concluded by stating, "By alleviating intestinal inflammation, [probiotic supplements] may act as a useful tool in the treatment of food allergy."[4] We'll explain later how to use probiotic supplements to restore your healthy gut bacteria and reduce your allergic potential.

Why Breast Milk Really Is Best

Not so long ago, every mother breast-fed her baby—as otherwise, the baby would die. Human breast milk is a treasure-house of essential nutrients and immune factors that help infants thrive naturally until they're ready to eat whole foods on their own. But as breast-feeding has declined during the past century, the prevalence of childhood allergies has increased dramatically.

The scientific literature stretching back over the last thirty years is clear. It strongly suggests that exclusive breast-feeding during the first four to six months of life delays by years the appearance and likelihood of food allergies, including:

- Otitis media (middle ear infection and fluid in the middle ear)

- Celiac disease (gluten sensitivity)

- Wheezing illnesses, like asthma and chronic bronchitis

- Chronic diarrheal diseases

- Autoimmune diseases

So the bottom line is: if at all possible, exclusively breast-feed your baby for at least six months in order to prevent or delay the appearance of food allergies and associated diseases. The sad truth is that very few mothers are heeding this advice. In the United Kingdom, two out of three mothers introduce their children to solids before the age of four months. In the United States, two out of three mothers introduce solid foods before six months and quit breast-feeding their babies entirely at six months.

They may not realize that breast-feeding protects their own health as well as their babies' health. Research from China, published in the *American Journal of Epidemiology*, shows that women who breast-feed their babies for two years have 50 percent less incidence of breast cancer compared to women who breast-fed for only one to six months.[5] Breast-feeding also greatly reduces the chances of the mother developing inflammation of the breasts (mastitis), and of their babies developing chronic diarrhea (which can be dangerous or even fatal in young children) and respiratory infections.[6]

While breast-feeding is brilliant health insurance, the mother's diet obviously affects breast milk—and with it, the chances of her baby developing allergies. Breast-fed children of mothers who eat a diet high in saturated fats, for instance, have a 16 percent higher risk of developing allergies, says Dr. Ulla Hoppu from Finland, who studied 114 breast-fed babies.[7] Nearly a quarter of this group of infants became sensitized to common allergens by the age of one, most commonly to eggs, milk, wheat, and cats.

So how does breast milk do the job of protecting babies from allergy? It has been found that complex proteins and amino acids in breast milk are key to the task. If levels of the natural organic compounds spermine and spermidine are low in breast milk, the child fed on it will have an 80 percent chance of developing an allergy. Adding these compounds to formula feed also reduces risk of developing allergy.[8] Breast milk is also higher in brain-friendly phospholipids and omega-3 fats, as long as the mother is eating oily fish and eggs, and, if indicated, supplementing omega-3 fish oils. (Oily fish is an excellent source of omega-3 fats, as well as other key nutrients like NADH, taurine, zinc, selenium, and sterols; eggs are a superb source of choline, a key component of memory-enhancing acetylcholine and brain cell membrane phosphatidylcholine.) These fats are not only vital for the brain; they are also essential building materials for healthy gut membranes, which means fewer allergy-provoking food proteins can get through.

Are We Too Clean?

Paradoxically, an overemphasis on hygiene and a germ-free environment during infancy and early childhood may also contribute to food allergies later in life. According to several recent studies, there is growing scientific evidence that too much emphasis on cleanliness and sterile childhood environments may be associated with as high as a 225 percent increased risk of developing allergies.

So it seems that exposure to germs early on may bring a degree of protection from childhood and adult food allergies. Surveys have found that children with the highest incidence of infections during infancy or early childhood—that is, living in the least hygienic surroundings—have the lowest incidence of food and airborne allergies later on. If subsequent studies bear this out, we may have to reevaluate our obsession with the mop and bucket, and conclude that our kids may be, heaven forbid, too clean!

Antacids and Antibiotics—Bad Medicine?

A new study by Austrian researchers indicates that the frequent use of antacids may produce food allergies. The study, headed by Professor Erika Jensen-Jarolim at the University of Vienna, involved approximately 300 people and found that those given antacid pills started to develop food allergy symptoms, while those taking placebos did not. The scientists said that antacid medications may interfere with digestion, thereby causing food to enter one's intestines and bloodstream before it is fully broken down, and so triggering an attack.[9]

A similar effect was found in children given antibiotics early in life. Researchers from the Henry Ford Hospital in Detroit, Michigan, found that children who receive antibiotics within their first six months significantly increase their risk of developing allergies.[10] The researchers found that compared to children not given antibiotics in that time, these children were almost twice as likely to develop asthma, allergies to pets, ragweed, grass, and dust mites by the age of seven. The study also showed the youngsters were less susceptible to these effects if they lived with at least two dogs or cats in their first year.

The Gene Factor

You can inherit allergies—at least the immediate-onset IgE kind.[11] If both your parents have this kind of allergy, there is a 75 percent chance that you will, too. If only one parent has, your odds are a 30 to 40 percent chance.[12] Pregnant women who suffer from allergies have been found to be more likely to have babies who develop allergies and asthma, according to a five-year study funded by the British Lung Foundation and Asthma U.K. The researchers, however, found that it is possible to minimize that risk by reducing a woman's exposure to allergens while she is pregnant. Dr. Jill Warner, who headed the research at Southampton General Hospital, said: "Our research shows that mothers can influence whether their baby develops sensitization to allergies. Controlling the mothers' reactions to allergens, especially during the second and third trimesters of pregnancy, may well be the treatment of the future, alongside more established advice such as giving up smoking and cutting down on alcohol."

In addition, certain people are not genetically predisposed to tolerate certain foods in their diets. Celiac disease, for example, is much more common among the Irish, Finnish, northern Sardinians, and possibly Native Americans.

Don't Abuse Alcohol

Drinking alcohol can increase anyone's allergy risk because it makes the gut more leaky by irritating the digestive tract. Research conducted by the University of Western Australia's Asthma and Allergy Research Institute has identified that wine in particular can trigger asthma attacks. They found that among 366 asthma sufferers, 1 in 3 reported that alcoholic drink triggered asthma attacks. Such reports were more common from people using steroid drugs or inhalers. In wine, the culprits involved are often sulfites,[13] while yeast or salicylates may also play a part.

Cross-Reactions—When Sensitivities Link

Another contributor to food sensitivity is exposure to allergens drifting around in the atmosphere. For example, it is well known that when the pollen count is high, more people suffer from hay fever in polluted areas than in rural areas, despite the lower pollen counts in cities. Exposure to exhaust fumes is thought to make a pollen-allergic person more sensitive. Whether this is simply because his or her immune system is weakened from dealing with the pollution and therefore less able to cope with the additional pollen insult, or due to some kind of "cross-reaction," is not known. In the United States, where ragweed sensitivity is common, a cross-reaction with bananas has been reported. In other words, one sensitivity sensitizes you to another. Hay fever sufferers may develop cross-reactions involving pollen, wheat, and milk.

The emerging view, shared by an increasing number of allergy specialists, is that food sensitivity is a multifactor phenomenon possibly involving poor nutrition, breast-feeding, alcohol, stress, genetics, pollution, digestive problems, abuse/overuse of antibiotics and anti-inflammatory painkillers, and overexposure to certain foods. Removing the foods may help the immune system to recover, but other factors need to be dealt with for any major impact on long-term food allergy to be made.

Addiction to Problem Foods

One interesting finding among people with food allergies is that they often become hooked on the very food that causes a reaction. This can actually lead to bingeing on the foods that harm them most, and withrawal-like symptoms if they go too long without eating these foods (see Chapter 5 for more information). Many people describe these foods as making them feel drugged or dopey. In some cases, the foods induce a mild state of euphoria, or a tranquilizing, calming effect. For these people, the food in question can actually become a psychological escape mechanism and a way of dealing with uncomfortable situations. But why do some foods cause drug-like reactions?

When pain no longer serves a purpose as part of a survival mechanism, chemicals called endorphins are released. These are the body's natural painkillers, and they make you feel good. The way they do this is by binding to sites that turn off pain and turn on pleasant sensations. Opiates such as morphine are similar in chemical structure and bind to the same sites, which is why they suppress pain.

Endorphins, whether made by the body or taken as a drug, are peptides—small groups of amino acids bound together. When a protein you eat is digested, it becomes peptides and, if the digestion works well, peptides that are two or three amino acids in length. In the laboratory, morphine-like peptides have been made from wheat, milk, barley, and corn using human digestive enzymes. These peptides have been shown to bind to endorphin receptor sites. Preliminary research does seem to show that certain foods, most commonly wheat and milk, may induce a short-term positive feeling, even if, in the long term, they are causing health problems. In autistic children, milk and gluten morphine-like chemicals are usually found in the urine, indicating leaky gut problems.

So it seems that frequently, the foods that don't suit you are also the foods you "couldn't live without." And in the first few days of giving up a suspect food, you may in fact start feeling pretty rough before you feel better. Some things are addictive in their own right: sugar, alcohol, coffee, chocolate, and tea (especially Earl Grey, which also contains the addictive essential oil bergamot). You can react to these foods without being allergic. Wheat and milk could be added to this list on the basis of their morphine-like effects.

REVERSING IgG FOOD ALLERGIES

Now you know all the major factors that, if solved, minimize your chances of developing allergies. Some you can act on now. Others, such as whether you were breast-fed or have a genetic legacy to deal with, are beyond your control. But the real trick to reversing your allergic tendency and losing your IgG allergies lies in two golden rules:

- Strictly avoid what you are allergic to.

- Heal your gut.

Simply Avoid It

What location is to a property that is for sale, strict elimination of allergic foods is to treating food allergy. Eliminating allergic foods means exactly that. Find out what you are allergic to by having an IgG food allergy test, and then strictly avoid your allergy foods for three to six months. This will demand very careful reading of labels on cans and packages, and exercising caution in restaurants.

The reason for the three to six months is that the IgG antibodies have a "half-life" of six weeks. This means that after six weeks, half of your IgG antibodies have died and been replaced, and after twelve weeks another half have died and been replaced. After three to six months you no longer have any of the IgG antibodies you had to start with. Provided you've been avoiding the foods you're allergic to, the new IgG antibodies inside you will no longer react to your food allergen if you reintroduce it.

Caveat: This does not apply to IgE-based, immediate-onset food allergies or to celiac disease. As far as we know, the only cure is lifelong avoidance of the food, although the anti-allergy diet and supplements we recommend may reduce your degree of allergic sensitivity here.

Heal the Gut

There are several possible underlying reasons why a person becomes food allergic. We've investigated a number of them: a lack of digestive enzymes, leaky gut, frequent exposure to alcohol or food containing irritant chemicals, immune deficiency leading to hypersensitivity of the immune system, and no doubt many more. Fortunately, tests exist to identify deficiencies in digestive enzymes, the "leaky gut syndrome," and the balance of bacteria and yeast in the gut. The tests can be arranged through qualified health professionals. To find one in your area, please see the Resources section at the back of this book.

There is a lot you can do to allow the gut and immune system to calm down and your allergic potential to decrease:

- Take digestive enzyme complexes (lipase, amylase, and protease) that help digest fat, protein, and carbohydrate. Since stomach acid and protein-digesting enzymes rely on zinc and vitamin B_6, it may help to take 15 milligrams (mg) of zinc and 50 mg of B_6 twice a day, as well as the digestive enzyme with each meal.

- Help heal your leaky gut. Cell membranes are made out of fat-like compounds, and one fatty acid—butyric acid—helps to heal the gut wall. The ideal daily dose is 1,200 mg. Vitamin A is also crucial for producing protective antibodies and for the health of any mucous membrane, including the gut wall, and taking 4–6 grams of powdered glutamine (an amino acid) in water before bed is also an excellent aid in helping the gut heal.

- Beneficial bacteria such as *Lactobacillus acidophilus* or *Bifidobacteria* can also help to calm down a reactive digestive tract.

- Boosting your immune system reduces any hypersensitivity it may have developed. Antioxidant nutrients and foods, glutamine, N-acetyl cysteine (NAC), vitamin A, B vitamins, zinc, thymic extract, and selenium all help to do this.

We look more closely at the foods, herbs, and nutrients that will help you fight food allergy below. And in Chapter 9, we put it all together: we'll tell you exactly what to eat and what to supplement in our 30-day digestive healing regime.

ANTI-ALLERGY FOODS, HERBS, AND NUTRIENTS

There are specific anti-allergy and anti-inflammatory foods, nutrients, and herbs that help to calm a hyped-up immune system. Let's take a look at these because each one is a vital piece of your action plan for food allergy relief, explained in Chapter 9.

Cornucopia of Health—Fruits and Vegetables

The more fresh fruits and vegetables you eat, the lower your risk of allergy. Specifically, apples and oranges have been shown to reduce the incidence of asthma symptoms.[14-15] Red onions and apples are especially high in quercetin (more on this powerful anti-allergy phytonutrient later).

Both fruit and vegetables are high in antioxidant nutrients that help calm down allergic reactions. Among these, vitamin C and quercetin are among the most powerful, and ones we recommend you also supplement (see Chapter 9). Onions and garlic contain the sulfur-rich amino acids cysteine and methionine, which help reduce allergic potential. It's also better to eat organic—not only because you do actually get more of these nutrients in organic produce, but also because that way you don't get exposed to a wide variety of toxic chemicals that can induce allergy in their own right.

The Essential Fats—Omega-3s and Omega-6s

The last three decades have seen a dramatic increase in the prevalence of asthma, eczema, otitis media, ADHD, allergic rhinitis, and many other allergy-related conditions. In parallel with this increase in allergy, there has been a decrease in the amounts of omega-3 fatty acids and an overall imbalance between all the essential fats we are getting in our diets. Omega-3s are essential fatty acids found most abundantly in oily fish and flaxseeds (also called linseeds). A true superfood, they protect our cells, promote brain health, balance our hormones, and reduce inflammation—which is why they're important in treating allergies.

But many people are failing to get the message. Along with the decline in omega-3 consumption there has been an upswing in the amount of vegetable and seed oils (along with animal fat, the so-called omega-6 fatty acids)—in margarine, for instance—we're eating. The vegetable and seed oils used in processed foods are especially bad news because the omega-6 fats they contain become damaged, and promote inflammation in the body. Some seed oils, like cottonseed oil, just shouldn't be eaten. For most people, the imbalance caused by eating much more omega-6s than omega-3s is unhealthy, too, as it can lead to overproduction of chemical troublemakers called inflammatory prostaglandins and leukotrienes, which make you more prone to chronic inflammation and allergies.[16]

In a study published in the *Medical Journal of Australia,* children who regularly ate fresh, oily fish had a significantly reduced risk of and protection from asthma. No other food groups or nutrients were associated with either an increased or reduced risk.[17] This is thought to be because a diet with a proper ratio between omega-3 and omega-6 fats makes you less likely to produce IgE antibodies and become allergic.[18] (According to many fatty acid researchers—and recently acknowledged by the World Health Organization—the proper ratio is four parts omega-6 to one part omega-3. Most Americans consume twenty-five times more omega-6 fats than omega-3s. This imbalance makes you prone to many diseases, including allergies.) So by eating more fresh, oily fish and other sources of omega-3 oils, you can reduce your allergic potential.

Flaxseeds and their oil are an acceptable omega-3 option, particularly for vegetarians. The ancient Greek physician and "father of medicine" Hippocrates wrote of using flaxseed for the relief of abdominal pain. And the greatest of all medieval kings, Charlemagne, considered flaxseed so healthy that he passed laws requiring its consumption. Along with its high omega-3 content, flaxseed is also very rich in fiber and lignans. Lignans are phytoestrogens (plant substances that mimic the action of the hormone estrogen) that are thought to bind to estrogen receptors in the body, and may have a role in preventing hormonally related cancers of the breast, uterus lining, and prostate gland. Although lignans are found in most unrefined grains (barley, buckwheat, millet, and oats), soybeans and some vegetables (broccoli, carrots, cauliflower, and spinach), flaxseed is the richest source.

Flaxseed contains both soluble and insoluble fiber (about 28 grams total fiber per 100 grams of flaxseed). About a third of the fiber is soluble. Studies have found that the soluble fiber in flaxseed—like that found in oat bran and fruit pectin—can help lower cholesterol and regulate blood sugar. The remaining two-thirds of the fiber in flaxseed is insoluble, which aids digestion by increasing bulk, reducing the time that waste remains in the body and preventing constipation.

Incorporating flaxseed into a diet is simple and can add a tasty twist to routine foods and dishes. The small, reddish-brown whole seeds have a nutty taste and can be sprinkled over salads, soups, yogurt, or cereals; grinding them will make the omega-3s more available. Whole or ground flaxseed can replace some of the flour in bread, muffin, pancake, and biscuit recipes. Flaxseed oil is also readily available in health food stores and may be substituted for other oils; ensure you keep it in the fridge to prevent it from going rancid.

So it makes good food-allergy-fighting sense to eat grilled or poached (never fried or breaded) wild or organic salmon, trout, orange roughy, cod, flounder, mackerel, sardines, herring, or other oily fish, accompanied by a bountiful mixed salad dressed with cold-pressed flaxseed oil. If you're vegetarian, go for walnuts, pumpkin seeds, sesame seeds, and omega-3-enriched eggs in addition to flaxseeds.

MSM—The Magic Molecule

MSM (methylsulfonylmethane) is a nontoxic, natural component of the plants and animals we eat and is also normally found in breast milk. This magic molecule contains a highly usable form of sulfur, the fourth most abundant mineral in the human body and part of the chemical makeup of over 150 compounds (all the proteins, as well as sulfur-containing amino acids, antibodies, collagen, skin, nails, insulin, growth hormone, and the most potent antioxidant, the enzyme glutathione). Vegans and people on a high-carbohydrate, low-protein diet probably don't get enough MSM. Antibiotic overuse may also contribute to sulfur deficiency by killing off the intestinal bacteria needed to produce essential sulfur-containing amino acids such as cysteine, taurine, and methionine.

Correcting a deficiency is important, as MSM has a number of proven benefits:

- It alleviates allergic responses to food and pollen allergens. The anti-allergic property of MSM is reported to be on a par with or better than traditional antihistaminic drugs.

- It provides relief for migraine headache sufferers.

- Daily supplementation is reported to provide dramatic and long-lasting relief of rheumatoid arthritis pain.

- It helps prevent and reverse the constipation seen in people with IBS and cow's milk allergy.

- It helps relieve snoring, a common food allergy symptom.

- Acne, acne rosacea, and diverse other skin problems associated with a leaky gut and food allergy respond favorably to MSM supplementation.

- It is particularly helpful for people experiencing allergy-related pain, stiffness, and swelling.

MSM appears to relieve allergies in a number of ways. It binds to or coats the lining of the small intestine, which may help soothe inflammation and reverse a leaky gut. MSM also provides the intestinal bacteria with building blocks for the manufacture of major anti-allergy, anti-inflammatory sulfur-containing amino acids, such as methionine and cysteine. Cysteine goes on to increase the production of glutathione, low levels of which are associated with an increased risk of premature death from all causes.

MSM is as safe as drinking water, and the daily therapeutic dose ranges from 1,000 to 6,000 mg. It works better if taken with vitamin C. Bear in mind that MSM is not like an aspirin or a shot of cortisol. A single, one-time dose of it is rarely effective in lessening symptoms. Reduction in pain, inflammation, and other allergic symptoms are usually seen within two to twenty-one days.

Glutamine—Fuelling Immunity

L-glutamine is an amino acid, literally the most abundant in the human body. It is the most important food or fuel for the small intestinal mucosa and the immune system. Like the MSM-derived amino acid, cysteine, glutamine is critical in maintaining optimal levels of the detoxifying, life-protecting antioxidant enzyme glutathione.

When in ample supply—that is, when you're well and not overly stressed from food allergies, celiac disease, Crohn's disease, ulcerative colitis, or chronic inflammation, or recovering from a major injury or excessive exercise—glutamine is able to quickly heal an inflamed intestine and maintain a healthy intestinal lining and immune system. If, on the other hand, you are chronically stressed from any physical or emotional cause, including food allergy, leaky gut, and a suppressed immune system, you will also be suffering from glutamine deficiency and will benefit from glutamine supplementation.

Taking glutamine has proven therapeutic benefits:

- It increases glutathione production in the liver, lymph nodes, intestinal lining, brain, and airways. This helps the food-allergy sufferer clear free radicals and immune complexes (see page 15) from circulation.

- It helps prevent and reverse leaky gut, including celiac disease, Crohn's disease, and ulcerative colitis.

- It helps prevent intestinal bleeding and ulceration in patients taking aspirin and other nonsteroidal anti-inflammatory drugs (NSAIDs) for food allergy-induced chronic pain syndromes such as arthritis, migraines, and fibromyalgia. In Japan, patients taking NSAIDs for pain and inflammation are instructed to take 2 grams of L-glutamine thirty minutes beforehand to prevent stomach bleeding and ulceration.

- It helps prevent or reverse poor nutrient status in food allergy patients experiencing malabsorption of nutrients.

- It helps prevent and heal peptic ulcers, a condition worsened by food allergy.

• It converts into GABA, a brain chemical associated with a calming, tranquilizing, anti-anxiety effect.

To get the best results with glutamine, you'll need to take 4 grams of glutamine powder—roughly 1 rounded teaspoon—dissolved in an 8-ounce glass of water, two or three times a day.

Anti-Allergy Antioxidants

Aside from their general role in keeping you optimally nourished, a number of key vitamins and minerals will help reduce your allergic potential.

Vitamin A

Vitamin A is an extremely important antioxidant and immune system-enhancing vitamin. Signs of deficiency include mouth ulcers, poor night vision, and skin problems such as acne. Here are some of its allergy-busting functions in the body:

• It maintains health of the mucous membranes and skin. Helpful in the prevention and treatment of eczema, psoriasis, and acne.

• As an antioxidant, it disarms highly destructive molecules, or free radicals, released during allergic reactions.

• It maintains a healthy thymus gland, the master gland of the immune system.

• It helps prevent the release of excessive inflammatory prostaglandins during allergic reactions.

• Along with zinc and probiotics, it helps in the production of two substances playing an important role in the digestive tract—protective mucus, and secretory IgA, which prevents bacteria, yeast, parasites, and food allergens from contacting the intestinal lining and passing into the bloodstream.

Vitamin A is of therapeutic value in the treatment of asthma, IBS, eczema, rheumatoid arthritis, and other food allergy-related disorders. Except for women who have not reached menopause, a basic dose of 6,000 micrograms (mcg) a day is very safe for most adults, and 3,000 mcg is minimal. Premenopausal women should not take more than 1,500 mcg of vitamin A a day because too much of this vitamin is associated with a potentially increased risk of birth defects. Also, as with all fat-soluble vitamins, there is the possibility of toxicity from overdoses of vitamin A.

Your individual tolerance level will depend on your metabolism, and general state of health. Signs that you are taking too much vitamin A can be dry skin, irritability, tenderness, or aching in the long bones of the body, headaches, cracking at the edges of the lips, hair thinning or loss, and abnormal liver function tests. Stop taking it to relieve the signs and symptoms. Recognizing the possible side effects of vitamin A supplementation, however, should not scare you away from including substantial amounts of this vital anti-allergy supplement in your daily regime.

Vitamin B₆

Vitamin B_6, in addition to being a major antioxidant, plays a big part in the metabolism of essential fatty acids into prostaglandins, and therefore has far-reaching effects on the cardiovascular, digestive, neurological, and immune systems. This vitamin is also linked to learning, behavioral, emotional, and mental processes, and plays a critical cofactor role in the production of brain neurotransmitters, including serotonin, which plays a key role in chronic pain, alcoholism, attention deficit hyperactivity disorder, sugar cravings, insomnia, depression, bipolar disorder, irritability, violence, and sexual promiscuity; GABA, nature's best antianxiety, stress-reducing brain chemical; and dopamine, important in mental alertness, energy, and pleasure. Some of the signs, symptoms, and medical conditions associated with B_6 deficiency include depression, anxiety, alcoholism and alcohol abuse, insomnia, inability to remember dreams, irritability and agitation, chronic fatigue or tiredness, wheezing and shortness of breath of asthma, old age, premenstrual syndrome, nausea and vomiting of pregnancy, morning sickness associated with oral contraception, recurring calcium oxalate kidney stones, hip fractures (hip fracture victims have very low B_6 levels), anemia, and eating disorders (bulimia and anorexia nervosa). Note, 38 percent of adult vegetarians are B_6 deficient.

Vitamin B_6 affects food allergies in a number of ways:

• It improves the production and release of hydrochloric acid in the stomach. Food allergy sufferers often don't produce enough stomach acid, probably because of food-allergy-induced gut hormone inhibition and malnutrition. B_6 works better when taken in conjunction with niacin (B_3), zinc, and a diet that eliminates food allergens.

• It helps relieve food allergy or gluten-induced psychological depression and ADHD-related hyperactivity.

• It helps in the treatment of certain forms of epilepsy and chronic pain syndromes.

- It stimulates the thymus gland, thereby contributing to the formation of antibodies and more optimally functioning immune cells.

B_6 deficiency is one of the most common nutrient deficiencies, yet the recommended dietary allowance (RDA) for this vitamin is pitifully low—just 2 mg a day. Many top nutritional scientists believe that a more optimal proper intake should be at least ten times this amount—20 mg. There are no safety concerns regarding amounts up to 200 mg a day.

Vitamin C

Vitamin C is a natural antihistamine, enhancing the action of the enzyme histaminase, which quickly breaks down histamine. That means it will give you instant relief during a histamine-based allergic reaction such as hay fever, as long as you take enough. One gram of vitamin C reduces blood histamine by approximately 20 percent, and 2 grams reduces histamine by over 30 percent.[19]

But there's much, much more to this phenomenal vitamin. C seems to be involved in almost all bodily functions. It is needed for the replacement of old tissue and the generation of new, making it invaluable for the healing of inflamed tissues and wounds. Healthy teeth and bones depend on its presence for strength and flexibility, as do the walls of capillaries and veins.

The vitamin's most profound effects, however, are in its overall strengthening of the immune system. It stimulates certain white blood cells, the phagocytes, to seek out and devour food allergens, bacteria, and viruses.

Vitamin C also acts as a powerful antioxidant, detoxifying many harmful free radicals, both in the environment and in the body, where these destructive molecules can be produced during allergic reactions. C is also known to reactivate both vitamin E, another powerful antioxidant, and the detoxifying, antioxidant, liver-protective enzyme glutathione. Asthmatics, especially those suffering from exercise-induced asthma, as well as hay fever sufferers and people with food-induced allergic rhinitis or arthritis, can benefit from the immune support provided by vitamin C.

If you're short on C, you may have bleeding gums, bruise easily, and catch frequent colds and infections.

Dr. Braly has also used large doses of vitamin C both orally and intravenously to detoxify and dramatically lessen chronic abstinence symptoms in recovering alcoholics, chemically dependant clients, and clients suffering from early withdrawals when eliminating food allergens from their diets.

How much C should you take? The minimum maintenance dose is 500 mg a day. The adult therapeutic dose begins at about 2,000 mg a day. As much as

8,000 to 16,000 mg daily, in divided doses, such as 2 grams every half-hour, may be indicated if you're having a severe allergic reaction; however, this is for short-term use only. Dr. Braly has used 25,000 mg of vitamin C intravenously to treat addictions. The most common reported side effect, even with these large amounts, is loose bowels.

It's a myth that vitamin C causes kidney stones. People with calcium oxalate kidney stones, which account for about 80 percent of all kidney stones, often lack magnesium and B_6. Supplementing these can help prevent calcium oxalate kidney stone formation.

Magnesium

Magnesium is the second most abundant mineral in the human body. It works closely with calcium and vitamin B_6 to regulate the heart, muscles, brain, and immune system. Research has shown that magnesium has a calming effect, working as a natural sedative—hence it's sometimes called the "antistress mineral."

Magnesium is also needed for essential fats to work properly, and plays a significant role in the prevention and treatment of various allergy-related conditions such as premenstrual syndrome, asthma, hyperactivity, autism, and migraine. During migraine attacks, an intravenous administration of 1 gram of magnesium has been shown to reverse the attack in over 80 percent of cases.[20-21] Magnesium supplements also help reduce symptoms of asthma, and intravenous magnesium at the time of an asthma attack has been shown to halve recovery time. If you're not getting enough, you may experience constipation, muscle cramps, migraine headaches, insomnia, depression, and irregular heartbeats.

We recommend taking 200 mg of elemental magnesium as a chelate (such as magnesium glycinate, citrate, or ascorbate) two to three times daily.

Zinc

Zinc has turned out to be far more influential in the treatment of food allergy than anyone thought. The mineral is a vital cofactor of essential fatty acid metabolism. Along with niacin and B_6, it is important for the production of hydrochloric acid in the stomach.

Zinc is a powerful immune-system stimulant.[22] It activates the thymus gland, which in turn produces the immune cell-stimulating hormone thymosin. Zinc is known to aid in restoring the delicate linings of the airways, and healing the gastrointestinal tract—in short, reversing a leaky gut. It also increases the levels of secretory immunoglobulin A (IgA) in the saliva and gut.

(Secretory IgA protects the gut by preventing bacteria, yeast, parasites, and food allergens from contacting the lining and passing into the bloodstream.) And it is needed for IgG antibody production.

Warning signs of a zinc deficiency include celiac disease, chronic inflammatory skin conditions, wounds that don't heal, poor dark/light adaptation, poor appetite, anorexia nervosa, retarded growth in a child, abnormal cravings for carbohydrates and sweets, impaired taste or smell, and frequent recurring infections. Many zinc deficient people also have visible white spots on their nail beds, and have low serum albumin and low normal alkaline phosphatase blood levels on routine blood chemistry tests.

Although the RDA for zinc is 15 mg per day, doses of 20 to 40 mg have had beneficial effects in conditions common among food allergy sufferers, such as acne, dermatitis herpetiformis (an extremely itchy rash associated with celiac disease), eczema, psoriasis, hyperactivity, eating disorders, and learning disabilities. Daily doses of 40 mg or higher should not be continued for longer than three months. Zinc depletes the body of copper. Therefore, it is recommended that 1 mg of copper should also be supplemented with every 10 to 15 mg of zinc.

Quercetin

The one daily supplement that often reduces allergic symptoms across the board is the phytonutrient quercetin, a chemical compound known as a bioflavonoid and found in plants. Sometimes, using just quercetin, a person can reintroduce allergen foods with no symptoms.

Quercetin is naturally found in wine, but not beer; tea, but not coffee; and the outer layers of red and yellow onions, but not white onions. Apples, lettuce, chives, berries, cherries, algae, and other plant materials also contain quercetin. The most studied, potent, and versatile of all 4,000 or so bioflavonoids, quercetin stabilizes mast cells in allergic patients. These mast cells, as we've seen, are unstable in allergy sufferers, and too readily release large quantities of histamine, inflammatory prostaglandins, cytokines, leukotrienes, and others of the chemical culprits behind allergic symptoms. Quercetin is also a potent antioxidant and anti-inflammatory agent.

For the best effect, quercetin should be taken in combination with vitamin C and a high-potency bromelain, the enzyme found in pineapple. For most people, the effective therapeutic dose is 500 mg of quercetin in combination with approximately 125 mg of high-potency bromelain and 250 to 500 mg vitamin C, taken thirty minutes before meals, two to three times a day. For maintenance (after your allergic symptoms have been brought under good control), reduce the above dose to once or twice daily, thirty minutes before breakfast and/or again before dinner.

Now we're ready to show you how to build all these and other anti-allergy foods, herbs, and nutrients into a powerful action plan for food allergy relief, using diet and supplements. We show you the ropes in the next chapter, including what to do for immediate relief if you have an allergic reaction.

Chapter 9

───◄○►───

Your Action Plan
for Food Allergy Relief

I
n this chapter we'll show you the most effective way to overcome your allergies by giving you the maximum chance of "unlearning" hidden food allergies and minimizing any reactions you do have.

It's important to note, however, that these techniques won't work if you have celiac disease, or immediate-onset allergies to foods like peanuts or shellfish, involving serious allergic reactions such as asthma or anaphylaxis. (We are assuming, by this stage, that you have found what you are allergic to by having an IgG food allergy test, a celiac screening test, and possibly an IgE food allergy test, too.) As far as we know, an immediate-onset IgE allergy means a permanent, fixed food hypersensitivity, and you must carefully avoid the allergen all your life.

However, in most cases, you can reverse—and even lose—delayed-onset IgG food allergies. Here's how you do it.

1. ELIMINATE YOUR FOOD ALLERGENS

There's no way around it: to treat an IgG food allergy, you need to start by strictly eliminating the allergen, and then rotating it with nonallergens (more on this soon). This means that for three to six months, you need to avoid that food—no ifs, ands, or buts.

For now, think in terms of three months minimum. You'll need to think beyond the obvious—read all the labels on cans and packages, question waiters in restaurants, anything to be sure of avoiding that particular food. If it's a favorite of yours, you'll need to be willing to give it up, and perhaps go through a few withdrawal or detoxification symptoms over the first three to five days. This may make you feel deprived—as if you miss a "good friend" who can temporarily make you feel better. But remember: it also means the end of allergic suffering and freedom from nagging, chronic, disabling physical, mental, and emotional symptoms. There's a good chance that you'll be feeling so fantastic at the end of our three-month program, you simply won't miss your allergic foods.

However, you'll need to be realistic from the start. Expect mild-to-moderate withdrawal or detoxification symptoms when coming off your allergens. Physiological addiction to food is no different from addiction to alcohol, caffeine, or tobacco. If you have allergies of a fairly severe nature, you can expect to go through a withdrawal period that usually lasts three to five days. The withdrawal symptoms usually reflect an intensification of symptoms you were already having, including headache, fatigue, poor sleep, anxiety, depression, irritability, stuffiness, joint aches, digestive upset, and severe food cravings. (One extremely effective treatment that helps prevent severe withdrawal is supplementing with large, therapeutic doses of vitamin C. Take 2 grams every hour, up to a maximum of 12 grams in one day, and continue for three consecutive days. If you get diarrhea during this time, halve the amount you take.)

2. EATS LOTS OF FRUIT AND VEGETABLES

As we learned in Chapter 8, eating lots of fruit and vegetables actually reduces your allergic potential, and gives you a great supply of antioxidants and other important nutrients. Whenever you can, eat organic, especially for foods you eat raw and unpeeled such as apples, pears, berries, tomatoes, and raw carrots. Make sure you always have a big bowl full of delicious fruit and vegetables for you and your family to snack on. Have something raw with most meals.

Many fruits and vegetables are also high in the anti-allergy nutrient quercetin. This not only acts as an anti-inflammatory, calming down any reactions that you have. It also calms down the immune system's mast cells (which release allergy-causing chemicals such as histamine), thereby reducing your allergic potential.

As you'll see from Table 9.1, the best vegetables for quercetin are, by a long way, red onions, followed by spinach, carrots, and broccoli. The best commonly available fruits to go for are apples and berries, especially cranberries and blueberries (red grapes are high in glucose, which can have a disruptive effect on blood sugar balance). We recommend you aim for at least 10 milligrams (mg) a day, although the more you take in from your diet the better. Table 9.1 shows you what that means in terms of what you eat. If you are a coffee drinker, think of changing to quercetin-rich tea.

3. GO FISHIN'

By now, we've seen how a diet high in omega-3 fish oils reduces your allergic

| TABLE 9.1. SOURCES OF QUERCETIN | | | |
FOOD	QUERCETIN (MG) PER 100 G FOOD	FOOD	QUERCETIN (MG) PER 100 G FOOD
Red onions	19.93	Sweet cherries	1.25
Cranberries	14.02	Plums	1.20
Spinach	4.86	Blackberries	1.03
Apples	4.42	Raspberries	0.83
Red grapes	3.54	Green peppers	0.65
Carrots	3.50	Strawberries	0.65
Broccoli	3.21	Tomatoes	0.57
Blueberries	3.11	Pears	0.42
Lettuce	2.47		

tendency. While a small number of people are allergic to white fish like cod, few are allergic to the oily fish such as salmon, mackerel, herring, sardines, and tuna, which are the best source of omega-3 fats. Basically, fish that eat fish tend to be highest in omega-3. There are also other very important nutrients found in fish, in addition to the oils, that may prove helpful in preventing and relieving many of the symptoms of food allergy. They include zinc, selenium, sterols, and NADH, a substance synthesized from niacin (vitamin B$_3$) that's contained in all living cells. NADH has been used clinically in the successful treatment of depression, ADHD, chronic fatigue, addictions, and Parkinson's disease. However, very large fish like swordfish, shark, kingfish (king mackerel), and albacore tuna can have substantial amounts of mercury in them, as this accumulates, too. Farmed fish are often loaded with antibiotics and pesticides, and due to feeding the farmed fish soybeans, may have only one-third the amount of omega-3 oils as "wild caught" (non-farmed) fish. So eat wild salmon or smaller oily fish as much as possible, aiming for two to three times a week.

4. EASY ON GRAINS AND DAIRY

Enough has been said and proven about the dangers of a diet high in dairy and gluten, or at least gliadin grains. So, go easy on wheat in particular and vary your diet so it isn't dependent on grains every day. Eat non-gliadin oats, and non-gluten grains such as buckwheat, rice, quinoa, amaranth, corn, millet, and teff. Vary your diet as much as possible, and don't eat the same foods every day.

5. ROTATE YOUR FOODS

Working out a new pattern to your eating so you're not consuming the same foods every day is—after avoiding allergens and healing a leaky gut—the single most important thing you can do to reverse and prevent a recurrence of food allergy.

Most food allergy tests will identify the foods you need to avoid (because they cause a significant antibody reaction) and foods that you can rotate (because they cause very little or no antibody reaction). If your allergy test result form doesn't specify foods to rotate, you can apply this principle to everything you eat, and certainly any of the foods in the top twenty food allergens listed in Chapter 6. In practice, what rotating will mean is that you will only eat that food once every three to four days—and preferably, less frequently.

So for at least the first three months following the complete elimination of all your food allergens, carefully rotate either those your food allergy test or health professional has advised you to rotate or, if you don't have this information, the top twenty food allergens. Rotating foods in this way really takes a load off your immune system and increases your chances of being able to reintroduce most of your allergens back into your daily diet—without allergic symptoms.

After three months, the principles of food rotation should still guide what and how you eat, though on a much more flexible basis. Nevertheless, the principles of rotation are the foundation of an allergy-free life. Here's why:

- A rotation diet helps prevent the development of allergies and thus a maladaptation to stress, called addiction. Food allergies develop for a wide variety of reasons, but a major one seems to be too frequent and/or too large an exposure to a potential food allergen, especially in the context of a leaky gut. (Our Stone Age ancestors, who had the same genetic makeup as us, were forced by seasons and scarcity to rotate and vary their foods.)

- Rotation encourages a more balanced, unprocessed, and varied and nutrient-dense diet and therefore leads to consuming more needed nutrients. If you are not going to repeat foods more often than every three days, you will have to get out of your eating rut! Most people's diets are dominated, calorie-wise, by no more than ten foods and sweetened and/or caffeinated beverages, ingested almost every day of their lives.

- Rotation dictates a simple, unrefined, additive-free diet. It is almost impossible to continue to eat processed, packaged foods on a rotation diet. Many packaged foods contain not one or two, but dozens of food ingredients, which, once eaten, cannot be eaten again for seventy-two to ninety-six hours if you're rotating your foods. The same goes for recipes with multiple ingredients and elaborate sauces or gravies.

- Rotation unstresses digestion. A rotation diet is what your digestive system was genetically designed to handle. Without overexposure to the same foods, food allergens, "bad" fats and oil, chemicals, additives, and excess refined sugar, your system can quickly strengthen and repair itself. Varied, nutrient- and fiber-rich, nonallergic foods bring about the optimal release of gut hormones and digestive juices; help heal and reverse an inflamed, leaky gut lining; improve absorption of nutrients; reduce toxic overload to the liver; and relieve constipation and diarrhea.

- *Food-allergen-free rotation quite often leads to dramatic weight loss— often without calorie counting or restriction of calories.* A rotation diet clears up the food allergies that lead to changes in brain chemistry, food cravings, overeating, a slowed metabolism, and water retention.

To plan a rotation diet, begin with a list of the foods to which you are not allergic. The next step is to plan three to four days of menus. Again, the meal plans should avoid all the foods to which you are allergic and should not repeat any nonallergic food for three or four days.

In this planning process, be guided by what you like (but not what you crave!), the time you have to prepare meals, and what is available at local supermarkets or health food stores. Keep it simple: use just a few foods and ingredients in each meal. If you have to avoid protein-rich foods like eggs, beef, and dairy products, make sure you get protein from alternative sources—nonallergenic fresh poached, baked, or grilled fish, turkey, chicken, or lentils and beans, for example. Here are some additional tips to make your rotation diet a success:

- Be an alert, smart shopper. Some common allergic foods show up in dozens of popular food items. That is why it is best to eat simple, fresh foods as much as possible.

- Avoid all alcohol for three months (booze of any kind is a major cause of a leaky gut).

- Have a big, fresh mixed vegetable salad every day; not eating enough fresh vegetables each day is a fundamental cause of allergy. Include quercetin-rich red or yellow onions, chives, and lettuce. The choice of salad dressing is important. Rotate your oils daily and select only unrefined, cold-pressed oils. Our preferences include cold-pressed flaxseed oil and extra virgin olive oil.

- Drink eight glasses of bottled or filtered water, and in addition, several cups of non-caffeinated herbal teas each day. Avoid fizzy or carbonated water. The carbon dioxide in the water converts it to an acidic liquid, making you more prone to chronic inflammations and allergies.

- If you have sleep problems, try not to eat or snack after 7 p.m. or so, and make the last meal of the day a lower-calorie, lower-animal protein, higher complex carbohydrate meal. Allow at least three hours between the end of your meal and bedtime. Food in the evening suppresses release of your sleep hormone, melatonin, preventing you from getting restful, healing, growth-hormone-releasing deep (stage 4) sleep.

- *There is no limit, except satisfaction of physiological hunger, on the amount that you eat. Do not count calories, do not remain hungry, and do not starve yourself. Concentrate on good nutrition and your health. If you're overweight, you'll be amazed when your weight begins to plummet without self-denial, and without counting a single calorie.*

Food families also need to be considered when you plan your rotation diet, since it is possible for a cross-reaction to occur to close relatives of foods you have an intolerance for. Foods from any one food family (see Appendix 1) should be eaten on the same day and, where possible, not eaten again for the next three days.

For example, if your food allergy test advises you to rotate cow's milk, rice, wheat, pea, salmon, pork, soybeans, and yeast, Table 9.2 gives an example of how to do it, with the food family shown in (*italics*).

TABLE 9.2. SAMPLE FOOD-ROTATION DIET			
DAY 1	**DAY 2**	**DAY 3**	**DAY 4**
Wheat (*grass*)	Wild salmon	Pea (*legume*)	Lean pork
Rice (*grass*)	Yeast	Soy (*legume*)	Cow's milk

HOW TO REINTRODUCE FOODS

Anyone who finds they have food allergies inevitably will ask the question, "Will I ever be able to eat the food(s) again?" After eliminating allergy-provoking foods for at least three months, and preferably six, most people with delayed food allergies find they can "clear" most of their food allergies. If done cautiously, one food at a time, you will be able reintroduce most of your formerly allergic foods back into your diet without allergic symptoms. Then, the chances are you will remain allergy-free, provided you continue to avoid the mistakes and bad dietary choices that led to food allergy in the first place.

On the other hand, life is not always fair. As we've said, people with celiac disease (gluten allergy) or with severe IgE allergies to peanuts or shellfish and symptoms such as anaphylaxis, asthma, or severe angioedema will have to carry syringes of adrenaline and antihistamine medication with them at all times. Needless to say, their respective allergens must also be carefully avoided for a lifetime.

Otherwise, here's how you go about reintroducing a food. After three months of strict rotation, reintroduce a moderate serving of previously offending foods back into your diet, one food at a time, every three days. If you're still allergic to certain foods, the three days allows time for delayed food allergic reactions to occur (recall that delayed reactions to foods normally appear between two hours and seventy-two hours after eaten).

Depending on your allergies, here are the best foods for you to reintroduce, and guidelines to make the reintroduction of foods most effective:

- If dairy has been avoided then a plain "bio-live" yogurt is the best to test first. If no reactions occur over a five-day period, try whole or half-and-half cow's milk. Avoid nonfat or low-fat milk initially due to its higher allergenicity.

- If wheat has been avoided, try a wheat-only product such as shredded wheat. Likewise, with oats, make a porridge of oats with water so it is only the oats themselves you are testing. The same is advisable with other grains.

- Egg is best tested by trying the cooked yolk only. If there is no reaction within five days then egg white could be tested next.

- When testing any of the foods choose a food made only of the product to be tested so you are positive it contains no other products.

- Always allow one week between reintroducing new foods. Any reaction and symptoms need to be monitored over the testing period.

- Reintroduce foods in ascending order of the severity of the reaction as given in your test results. So that means starting with the foods that gave the weakest reaction because your body is more likely to have forgotten about these foods first.

To make it easy for you, we've included a symptom score chart in Appendix 2 for you to use to record your symptoms as you reintroduce foods. In this way you can keep a clear record of what happens. If you do not react in three days, then it is likely that you can reintroduce this food into your diet, although we advise that you continue to rotate it and/or eat the food infrequently.

ANTI-ALLERGY SUPPLEMENTS

In addition to eliminating your food allergens and following a rotation diet, certain natural supplements can help you to recover more quickly from food allergies and decrease your allergic potential. We had a look at these in the previous chapter—now let's see how you put it into action.

Immune-Boosting Supplements

Your immune system depends on a minute-by-minute supply of a wide range of nutrients, especially vitamin A, B vitamins, zinc, magnesium, and selenium. In addition to eating a nutrient-rich, nonallergic whole-food diet we recommend that you supplement these nutrients on a daily basis.

Here are the kind of levels you want to supplement on a daily basis:

Vitamin A:	1,500 mcg	Vitamin B$_6$:	25 mg
Beta-carotene		Magnesium:	200 mg
(as mixed carotenoids):	500 mcg	Zinc:	15 mg

You can find all of these in a good high-strength multivitamin. The best multivitamin and mineral supplements recommend taking two a day, for the simple reason that you can't get all these ideal levels into one tablet or capsule.

Even so, you'll never find enough vitamin C in a multi, so this needs to be taken separately as well. We recommend anyone with allergies to supplement 1,000 mg twice a day and possibly more, especially if you are in the withdrawal phase or still experiencing allergic symptoms.

Anti-Allergy and Anti-Inflammatory Supplements

Vitamin C is the most important anti-allergy vitamin. It is a powerful promoter of a strong immune system, immediately calms down allergic reactions and is also anti-inflammatory. It's really recommended for every adult at an absolute minimum of 1,000 mg (1 g) a day, although 2,000 mg (2 g) or more is optimum for most people, whether or not you have allergies. If you are suffering from allergic symptoms, you might want to take twice this amount on a regular basis. Since vitamin C is in and out of the body within six hours, it's best taken in divided doses, either 1 gram in the morning and 1 gram at lunch or, if you are taking larger amounts, 1 gram four times a day. *Note:* If you have a history of recurring kidney stones, it is advisable that you take extra vitamin B$_6$ and magnesium, in a decent multivitamin for example, daily with your vitamin C.

Omega-3 fish oils are one of nature's best natural anti-inflammatory nutrients, with countless other benefits besides. Although you can and should obtain these from eating unfried, unbreaded fish, we recommend you supplement omega-3 fish oils every day as an insurance policy. To give you a rough idea, we recommend you take in the equivalent of 1,000 mg of combined EPA and DHA (these are the two most powerful omega-3 fatty acids) a day, or 7,000 mg a week. A 100 gram serving of mackerel might give you 2,000 mg, while a serving of salmon might give you 1,000 mg. So, if you eat fish three times a week you'll probably achieve 3,500 mg a week. To make up the remaining 3,500 mg we recommend you take an omega-3 fish oil supplement providing 500 mg of combined EPA and DHA a day. This is good advice for anyone, even if you're not especially allergic. *Warning:* Do not make the fundamental mistake of going overboard by severely restricting vegetable oils, seed oils, animal fats, butter, and egg yolk. You need all these essential oils in your diet daily, not just fish oil.

Quercetin, like omega-3 and vitamin C, is provided in the foods we recommend you eat, but you'll be hard pushed to eat more than 20 mg a day. That's good and to be highly recommended, but supplementing 500 mg three times a day when suffering from severe allergies and 500 mg a day once you have your allergies under control as a maintenance dose is effective for reducing allergic potential. The best results are achieved by supplementing 250 mg, twice a day, with some bromelain (digestive enzyme from pineapple) and vitamin C. Some quercetin supplements contain all these in one.

MSM has so many benefits for allergy sufferers that it's hard to know where to start. As long as you're still suffering from any allergic symptoms, or in pain, it's well worth supplementing MSM on a daily basis. While therapeutic intakes go up to 6,000 mg a day, we recommend you start with 1,000 mg twice a day.

Glutamine is an essential part of any regime designed to quickly restore a healthy digestive tract and prevent further damage from foods, alcohol, or anti-inflammatory, pain-relieving medications. It is also a powerful nutrient for supporting proper immune function and protecting the liver. For this reason, we not only recommend it as part of healing a leaky gut, but also for anyone during the first thirty days of following an action plan for food allergy relief. The ideal amount is 8 to 12 grams mixed and consumed in cold or warm (not hot) water each day. A well-rounded teaspoon is about 4 grams. So 2 to 3 rounded teaspoons a day is recommended. For best results, drink the glutamine solution on an empty stomach, on waking and before bed.

Each of these five nutrients is nontoxic and we highly recommend you take them for the first thirty days to rapidly reduce your allergic potential. If you find them particularly effective and wish to continue supplementing them on a regular basis, go ahead—you'll be doing your overall health a massive favor.

THE ACTION PLAN: A RECAP

In short, here's what to do to minimize your allergic potential and swiftly become allergy-free.

Your Anti-Allergy Diet

- Eliminate your food allergens. Read labels carefully.
- Follow a strict three- or four-day rotation diet.
- Minimize wheat and milk products even if you're not allergic.
- Have a large mixed salad every day and at least three portions of vegetables.
- Have two to three pieces of fruit every day.
- Consume at least 10 mg of quercetin each day from tea and foods such as red onions, apples, and berries, although you'll benefit from more in supplements.
- Eat unfried, unbreaded oily fish rich in omega-3 fats—such as mackerel, halibut, sardines, herring, orange roughy, or wild salmon—two or three times a week.
- Eat ground flaxseeds and pumpkin seeds, and use flaxseed oil and extra virgin olive oil in salad dressings.
- Drink eight glasses of water or herbal tea every day. Avoid fruit juices and other sweetened drinks.

YOUR PRESCRIPTION FOR HEALING THE GUT

Allergies and leaky gut syndrome is one of those chicken-or-egg situations. There's good reason to suppose that having a more permeable digestive tract is what precipitates food allergies in the first place, while having a food allergy encourages a leaky gut by inflaming the digestive tract wall. While you can test for increased gastrointestinal permeability, it's highly likely that you have a degree of increased permeability, especially if you have multiple food allergies or digestive symptoms. Since the digestive tract lining is rapidly replacing itself, here's what you can do in thirty days to quickly improve the health of your "inner skin," thereby reducing your allergic potential. These recommendations complement the diet and supplement action points discussed above, rather than replacing them:

Digestive enzymes that help digest fat, protein, and carbohydrate—that

Your Anti-Allergy Supplements		
	A.M.	**P.M.**
Every day		
• High-strength multivitamin	1	1
• Vitamin C 1,000 mg	1	1
• Omega-3 fish oils (500 mg of EPA/DHA)	1	1
For the first 30 days (otherwise optional)		
• Quercetin 500 mg+	1	1
• MSM 1,000 mg	1	1
• Glutamine powder (1 teaspoon = 4 g)	1 tsp	1 tsp
Additional nutrients for healing a leaky gut		
• Digestive enzymes	1 with each meal	
• Probiotics (*Lactobacillus, Bifidobacteria*) plus prebiotics such as FOS	1 with each meal	
• Butyric acid or caprylic acid 350 mg	1 with each meal	

Unless otherwise stated, take nutritional supplements with food. Glutamine powder is best taken in water on an empty stomach, first thing in the morning and/or last thing at night. Occasionally, some people find glutamine too energizing if taken last thing at night.

is, lipase, amylase, and protease—are well worth trying if you have any digestive problems or food allergy symptoms. Since stomach acid and protein-digesting enzymes rely on zinc and vitamin B_6, it may help to take 15 mg of zinc and 50 mg of B_6 twice a day, as well as a digestive enzyme with each meal.

Butyric acid or caprylic acid are medium-chain triglycerides (blood fats) and help to heal the gut wall, partly because the membranes of intestinal cells are largely made out of such fats. The ideal daily dose of either is 900 mg to 1,200 mg a day, or 300 mg to 400 mg three times a day.

Probiotics such as *Lactobacillus* and *Bifidobacteria* taken together can also help to calm down a reactive digestive tract and reduce allergic potential. Probiotic bacteria need to eat to survive. This is where "prebiotics" come into play. Prebiotics are nondigestible, fermentable food ingredients that feed and stimulate friendly bacteria in the intestines. They increase the densities of ben-

PS: WHAT TO DO IF YOU'VE HAD AN ALLERGIC REACTION

If you are having an allergic reaction and want to recover as quickly as possible, here's what to do until the allergic symptoms subside:

- Stop eating!

- Drink only filtered water and drink plenty of it (at least ten glasses of water during the day). A measure that you are drinking enough is that you'll have to urinate frequently, and that the urine will be clear.

- Begin taking large therapeutic doses of crystal vitamin C (as ascorbic acid). Take 1 rounded teaspoon of vitamin C (about 2 to 4 g) every thirty to sixty minutes until it causes watery stools—not loose stools, but diarrhea. This may take eight to twenty-four hours. Then, reduce to $\frac{1}{2}$ teaspoon every hour until the symptoms are gone. (*Note:* If you have a history of recurring kidney stones, you should also be taking 400 mg of magnesium and 50 mg of vitamin B_6 daily during this time.)

- When your allergic symptoms are gone and you begin eating again, be extremely careful to avoid all the foods you were eating during the three days before the onset of your allergic reaction. And eat much smaller portions of all foods for several days, chewing the foods thoroughly without swallowing until they become a liquid slurry. Otherwise, you may react again!

eficial bacteria and stimulate growth and functions of the healthy intestine. Recent findings show that after acute diarrhea, giving a prebiotic accelerates recovery of beneficial bacteria, reduces the relative abundance of detrimental, disease-causing bacteria, stimulates intestinal mucosal growth, and enhances digestion and immunity. Prebiotics are often included in probiotic supplements for this reason. Examples of prebiotics include fructooligosaccharides (FOS), inulin (from fermentable chicory fructan, a kind of carbohydrate), guar gum, and pectin. Look out for probiotic supplements containing these as well as a billion or more viable organisms, providing both *Lactobacillus* and *Bifidobacteria.*

Appendix 1

—◄◦►—

Know Your Food Families

As they're all based on plants or animals, foods can be grouped into families depending on which ones they're derived from, and many will share similar proteins, and hence similar potential allergens, with their close relatives. It's well worth knowing these food families. For example, both cashew nuts and pistachios are from the *cashew* family. This means that if you react to one, you are more likely to react to the other. *Crustaceans*—crab, crayfish, lobster, prawn, and shrimp—are quite different from *mollusks,* which include abalone, clams, mussels, oysters, scallops, snails, and squid. *Octopus* is in a family of its own. If you react to crustaceans, there is no reason why you should react to mollusk or octopus family foods.

FOOD BY FAMILY NAME	
FAMILY NAME	FOODS IN THE FAMILY
Plants	
Banana	Arrowroot, banana, ginger, plantain, turmeric, vanilla
Beech	Beechnut, chestnut
Beet	Beet, chard, spinach, sugar beet
Berry	Blackberry, boysenberry, loganberry, raspberry, strawberry
Birch	Hazelnut, wintergreen
Buckwheat	Buckwheat, rhubarb, sorrel
Carrot	Angelica, caraway, carrot, celery, chervil, coriander, cumin, dill, fennel, parsley, parsnip
Cashew	Cashew nuts, mango, pistachio
Citrus	Citron, grapefruit, lemon, lime, mandarin, orange, tangerine
Composites	Artichoke, chamomile, chicory, dandelion, endive, lettuce, safflower, salsify, sunflower, tarragon

FAMILY NAME	FOODS IN THE FAMILY
Fungi	Mushrooms, truffle, yeast
Gourd	Cucumber, gherkin, melon (honeydew), pumpkin, squash, watermelon, zucchini
Grape	Grape, raisin, sultana, cream of tartar (a byproduct of winemaking)
Grass	Bamboo shoots, barley, corn, millet, oat, rice, rye, sorghum, sugar cane, wheat
Heather	Blueberry
Laurel	Avocado, bay leaf, cinnamon, sassafras
Legume	Bean, carob, lentil, licorice, pea, peanut, senna, soy, tapioca
Lily	Asparagus, chive, garlic, leek, onion, shallot
Madder	Coffee
Mint	Basil, bergamot, lavender, lemon balm, marjoram, mint, oregano, rosemary, sage, thyme
Mulberry	Breadfruit, fig, hop, mulberry
Mustard	Broccoli, Brussels sprouts, cabbage, cauliflower, Chinese leaves, cress, horseradish, kale, kohlrabi, mustard, radish, rapeseed, turnip, watercress
Olive	Olive
Palm	Coconut, date, palm, sago
Pineapple	Pineapple
Potato (nightshade family)	Cayenne pepper, chili pepper, eggplant, paprika, pepper, potato, sesame, tahini, tobacco, tomato
Rose	Apple (including cider), crab apple, pear, rosehip
Rosestone	Almond, apricot, cherry, nectarine, peach, plum, prune, quince, sloe
Saxifrage	Blackcurrant, currant, gooseberry
Stericula	Chocolate, cocoa, cola
Tea	Tea
Verbena	Lemon verbena
Walnut	Butternut, pecan nut, walnut
Poultry and Wildfowl	
Dove	Pigeon
Duck	Duck, goose
Grouse	Grouse, partridge

FAMILY NAME	FOODS IN THE FAMILY
Guinea fowl	Guinea fowl
Pheasant	Chicken (and their eggs), peafowl, pheasant, quail
Turkey	Turkey
Meat	
Bovid	Beef, beef dairy products (cow's milk, cream, casein/caseinate, whey, yogurt, cheese), buffalo, feta, gelatin, goat, goat's milk and cheese, lamb, sheep's milk and cheese, Roquefort, veal
Deer	Caribou, elk, moose, reindeer, venison
Hare	Hare, rabbit
Swine	Pork
Seafood	
Crustacean	Crab, crayfish, lobster, prawn, shrimp
Mollusk	Abalone, clam, cockle, mussel, oyster, scallop, snail, squid
Octopus	Octopus
Freshwater Fish	
Bass	Bass, perch (white), yellow bass
Herring	Shad
Minnow	Carp, chub
Perch	Perch (yellow), red snapper
Pike	Pickerel, pike
Salmon	Salmon, trout
Smelt	Smelt
Sturgeon	Caviar, sturgeon
Sunfish	Black bass
Saltwater Fish	
Anchovy	Anchovy
Codfish	Cod, cod liver oil, haddock, hake, pollack
Eel	Eel
Flounder	Flounder, halibut, plaice, sole, turbot
Mackerel	Bonito, mackerel, tuna
Mullet	Mullet
Porgy	Bream, porgy
Salmon	Salmon, sea trout

FAMILY NAME	FOODS IN THE FAMILY
Scorpion fish	Ocean perch, rockfish
Sea bass	Grouper, sea bass
Sea catfish	Catfish
Sea herring	Herring, pilchard, sardine
Skate	Skate
Honey	Honey contains multiple plant pollens, while commercial honey frequently contains sugar

FOOD FAMILIES BY INDIVIDUAL FOODS

FOOD ITEM	FAMILY	FOOD ITEM	FAMILY
Grains			
Barley	Grass	Rice	Grass
Buckwheat	Buckwheat	Rye	Grass
Corn (maize)	Grass	Sago	Palm
Malt	Grass	Tapioca	Grass
Millet	Grass	Wheat	Grass
Oat	Grass		
Dairy			
Brie	Bovid	Goat's milk	Bovid
Cheddar	Bovid	Gouda	Bovid
Cottage cheese	Bovid	Processed cheese	Bovid
Cow's milk	Bovid	Sheep's milk	Bovid
Edam	Bovid	Stilton	Bovid
Egg (whole)	Pheasant	Swiss cheese	Bovid
Evaporated milk	Bovid	Whey (cow's)	Bovid
Goat's cheese	Bovid	Yogurt	Bovid
Meat/Poultry			
Beef	Bovid	Pork	Swine
Chicken	Pheasant	Rabbit	Hare
Duck	Duck	Turkey	Turkey
Lamb	Bovid	Venison	Deer
Liver (beef)	Bovid		

Fish			
Anchovy	Anchovy	Plaice	Flounder
Clam	Mollusk	Prawn	Crustacean
Cod	Codfish	Salmon	Salmon
Crab	Crustacean	Sardine	Sea herring
Haddock	Codfish	Scallop	Mollusk
Halibut	Flounder	Skate	Skate
Mackerel	Mackerel	Sole	Flounder
Mussels	Mollusk	Trout	Salmon
Oyster	Mollusk	Tuna	Mackerel
Pilchard	Sea herring		

Vegetables			
Artichoke	Composite	Lentils	Legume
Asparagus	Lily	Lettuce	Composite
Avocado	Laurel	Mustard	Mustard
Bean sprouts	Legume	Onion	Lily
Beetroot	Beet	Parsnip	Carrot
Broccoli	Mustard	Pea	Legume
Brussels sprouts	Mustard	Pinto beans	Legume
Butterbeans	Legume	Potato	Potato
Cabbage	Mustard	Radish	Mustard
Carob	Legume	Rhubarb	Buckwheat
Carrot	Carrot	Safflower	Composite
Cauliflower	Mustard	Soybean	Legume
Celery	Carrot	Spinach	Beet
Chickpea	Legume	Squash	Gourd
Cucumber	Gourd	Sunflower	Composite
Eggplant	Potato	Sweet potato	Morning glory
Endive	Composite	Tomato	Potato
Green beans	Legume	Turnip	Mustard
Haricot beans	Legume	Yam	Yam
Kidney beans	Legume	Zucchini	Gourd
Leek	Lily		

FOOD ITEM	FAMILY	FOOD ITEM	FAMILY
Fruits			
Apple	Rose	Lemon	Citrus
Apricot	Rosestone	Lime	Citrus
Banana	Banana	Mango	Cashew
Blackberry	Berry	Melon	Gourd
Blackcurrant	Saxifrage	Olive	Olive
Blueberry	Heather	Orange	Citrus
Cherry	Rosestone	Peach	Rosestone
Date	Palm	Pear	Rose
Fig	Mulberry	Pineapple	Pineapple
Gooseberry	Saxifrage	Plum	Rosestone
Grape	Grape	Raspberry	Berry
Grapefruit	Citrus	Strawberry	Berry
Hops	Mulberry	Sultana	Grape
Kiwi	Kiwi		
Nuts			
Almond	Rosestone	Hazelnut	Birch
Brazil nut	Brazil	Peanut	Legume
Cashew nut	Cashew	Pecan nut	Walnut
Chestnut	Beech	Pistachio	Cashew
Coconut	Palm	Walnut	Walnut

Food Item	Family	Food Item	Family
Spices/Herbs			
Arrowroot	Banana	Nutmeg	Nutmeg
Basil	Mint	Oregano	Mint
Bay leaf	Laurel	Parsley	Carrot
Cayenne pepper	Potato	Pepper (black)	Peppercorn
Chicory	Composite	Pepper (white)	Peppercorn
Chili	Potato	Rosemary	Mint
Cinnamon	Laurel	Sage	Mint
Coriander	Carrot	Sesame seed	Potato
Fennel	Carrot	Tarragon	Composite
Garlic	Lily	Thyme	Mint
Ginger	Banana	Tobacco	Potato
Licorice	Legume	Turmeric	Banana
Mustard	Mustard	Vanilla	Banana
Others			
Beet sugar	Beet	Maple syrup	Maple
Cane sugar	Grass	Mushrooms	Fungi
Chamomile	Composite	Rapeseed	Mustard
Chocolate/cocoa	Stericula	Tea	Tea
Coffee	Madder	Yeast	Fungi
Cola	Stericula		

Appendix 2

---◄○►---

Symptom
Score Chart

The chart on the following pages is designed for people with IgG delayed-onset allergies who have cut their allergen foods out for three months and want to reintroduce those foods. If that's you, this chart will help you monitor that process.

We recommend that you keep a daily record of what you eat, any symptoms that you might be having (keeping in mind that a symptom you have today may have been caused by food you ate a day or two days before), and any other factor that might alter your progress. It is also advisable to keep a record of your weight, since rapid weight gain in one day (3 or more pounds) is a very frequent symptom of food allergy.

Note that we've devised a scoring system that you may find helpful when you're trying to gauge how each symptom is affecting you each day.

The scores are as follow:

    3 = very bad

    2 = bad

    1 = not too bad/improving

    0 = not a problem

DAY/DATE	SYMPTOMS AND SCORE	WEIGHT	NOTES
1			1st avoid food reintroduced
2			
3			
4			
5			
6			
7			
8			2nd avoid food reintroduced
9			
10			
11			
12			
13			
14			
15			3rd avoid food reintroduced
16			
17			
18			
19			
20			
21			

DAY/DATE	SYMPTOMS AND SCORE	WEIGHT	NOTES
22			4th avoid food reintroduced
23			
24			
25			
26			
27			
28			
29			5th avoid food reintroduced
30			
31			
32			
33			
34			
35			
36			6th avoid food reintroduced
37			
38			
39			
40			
41			
42			

DAY/DATE	SYMPTOMS AND SCORE	WEIGHT	NOTES
43			7th avoid food reintroduced
44			
45			
46			
47			
48			
49			
50			

Appendix 3

---◀◯▶---

Abstinence Symptom Severity Scale

Name: _____ **Date:** _____

Please circle the number that best indicates the severity of each symptom you are experiencing **today** *(zero indicates the absence of the symptom, 10 represents an extreme, intolerable intensity level).* **Answer each question as honestly and accurately as possible.**

Low Level										High Level

Craving or drug hunger

0   1   2   3   4   5   6   7   8   9   10

Craving for sweets/sugar/bread

0   1   2   3   4   5   6   7   8   9   10

Craving for salt

0   1   2   3   4   5   6   7   8   9   10

Loss of appetite

0   1   2   3   4   5   6   7   8   9   10

Overeating/always hungry

0   1   2   3   4   5   6   7   8   9   10

Bloating or sleepiness after eating

0   1   2   3   4   5   6   7   8   9   10

Sense of emptiness/incompleteness

0   1   2   3   4   5   6   7   8   9   10

Anxiety

0   1   2   3   4   5   6   7   8   9   10

Internal shakiness

0   1   2   3   4   5   6   7   8   9   10

Restlessness
| 0 | 1 | 2 | 3 | 4 | 5 | 6 | 7 | 8 | 9 | 10 |

Impulsiveness/act before thinking
| 0 | 1 | 2 | 3 | 4 | 5 | 6 | 7 | 8 | 9 | 10 |

Difficulty concentrating/focusing
| 0 | 1 | 2 | 3 | 4 | 5 | 6 | 7 | 8 | 9 | 10 |

Fuzzy thinking/head cloudy
| 0 | 1 | 2 | 3 | 4 | 5 | 6 | 7 | 8 | 9 | 10 |

Memory problems/memory loss
| 0 | 1 | 2 | 3 | 4 | 5 | 6 | 7 | 8 | 9 | 10 |

Depression
| 0 | 1 | 2 | 3 | 4 | 5 | 6 | 7 | 8 | 9 | 10 |

Mood swings
| 0 | 1 | 2 | 3 | 4 | 5 | 6 | 7 | 8 | 9 | 10 |

Negative self-talk
| 0 | 1 | 2 | 3 | 4 | 5 | 6 | 7 | 8 | 9 | 10 |

Irritability/impatience with people
| 0 | 1 | 2 | 3 | 4 | 5 | 6 | 7 | 8 | 9 | 10 |

Daytime sleepiness/drowsiness
| 0 | 1 | 2 | 3 | 4 | 5 | 6 | 7 | 8 | 9 | 10 |

Problems getting to or staying asleep
| 0 | 1 | 2 | 3 | 4 | 5 | 6 | 7 | 8 | 9 | 10 |

Fatigue/lack of energy/worn out
| 0 | 1 | 2 | 3 | 4 | 5 | 6 | 7 | 8 | 9 | 10 |

Hypersensitivity to stress
| 0 | 1 | 2 | 3 | 4 | 5 | 6 | 7 | 8 | 9 | 10 |

Hypersensitivity to sound or noise
| 0 | 1 | 2 | 3 | 4 | 5 | 6 | 7 | 8 | 9 | 10 |

Hypersensitivity to pain
| 0 | 1 | 2 | 3 | 4 | 5 | 6 | 7 | 8 | 9 | 10 |

Muscle or joint pain/headaches
| 0 | 1 | 2 | 3 | 4 | 5 | 6 | 7 | 8 | 9 | 10 |

Total score here: _____

Before IV/oral nutrient therapy total scores above 100 are common among recovering alcoholics and drug addicts. After one week of IV/oral therapy, most clients achieve and maintain total scores under 35, some under 10. Please refer to Chapter 5 for more information.

Appendix 4

⏤◇⏤

Celiac Disease

Celiac disease is a permanent, serious, inherited condition characterized by an allergic toxicity to gliadin—a glycoprotein (carbohydrate plus protein) found in gluten cereals (wheat, rye, and barley, as well as Kamut, spelt, and triticale). If people with this illness consume any gliadin (and it doesn't take much—less than half a gram), the gliadin will attack the lining of their intestines. The lining becomes leaky and loses its ability to absorb nutrients from food. Pronounced malabsorption and malnutrition set in, along with deficiencies in omega-6 and omega-3 essential fats, iron, zinc, calcium, magnesium, potassium, selenium, and vitamins B_1, B_6, B_{12}, folic acid, A, D, E, and K.

There is a strong genetic aspect to celiac disease. Seventy percent of identical twins both get it, making it 175 times more prevalent than in the general population—which points to a strong genetic tendency. If one of your parents or siblings has celiac disease, you have a one in ten chance of having it, too—or in other words, over ten times higher risk than the average person.

Medical textbooks may still say that it occurs in only 1 in 5,000 or so people. Due to remarkable advances in laboratory screening for celiac sufferers, we have learned that it occurs more frequently than anyone ever imagined. According to a random sampling by the American Red Cross, 1 in 250 people in the United States suffer from celiac disease—and nineteen out of every twenty cases still go undetected and untreated. More recent studies appearing in the top medical journal the *Lancet* have reported a prevalence of 1 in 250 Italians, 1 in 122 Irish, 1 in 111 healthy, asymptomatic Americans, 1 in 85 Finnish, 1 in 70 Italians in northern Sardinia,[1] and 1 in 18 Algerian Saharawi refugee children.

Celiac disease is thought to be such a health threat in Italy that the government at one time was considering mandating that all children, regardless of whether they are sick or not, must be tested for gliadin sensitivity and celiac disease by the age of six. In the United States and Britain we are still in the Dark Ages in terms of recognizing the widespread prevalence of celiac disease.

A SHIFT IN SIGNS AND SYMPTOMS

The other medical myth about celiac disease is that a doctor should be able to diagnose a patient easily through "unmistakable" abdominal and other traditional signs and symptoms: chronic diarrhea/episodic diarrhea with malnutrition, abdominal cramping, abdominal distention or bloating, foul-smelling, bulky stools (steatorrhea), weight loss or poor weight gain, short stature, iron-deficiency anemia, and a patient complaining of weakness, fatigue, and loss of appetite.

This scenario is changing irrevocably, however. Today, most people with undiagnosed celiac disease no longer go to the doctor complaining of abdominal problems. Instead, they could come through the door with a whole range of varied symptoms:

- Chronic psychological depression*
- Abnormal elevation of liver enzymes of unknown cause
- Permanent teeth with distinctive horizontal grooves and chalky whiteness
- Chronic nerve disease of unknown cause (such as ataxia or peripheral neuropathy)
- Osteoporosis in women not responding to conventional therapies
- Repeated low-impact bone fractures
- Intestinal cancers
- Insulin-dependent diabetes
- Thyroid disease (both overactive and underactive)
- Short stature in children
- Down's syndrome in children

*Some authorities say chronic psychological depression is the most common presenting symptom of celiac disease, especially if the depressed patient has not responded well to prescription antidepressant medications.

Undetected gluten sensitivity, whether or not it has led to celiac disease, is commonly found among pre- and postmenopausal women and even children who suffer from osteoporosis. The same nutrient deficiencies found in osteoporosis—magnesium, vitamin D, and vitamin K—are also seen in people suffering from celiac disease. In fact, one recent study showed that a gluten-free diet actually reversed osteoporosis in people with celiac disease. They took 44 celiac patients aged from two to twenty at the time of their diagnosis, and compared them with 177 healthy, celiac-free people. The lumbar spine and whole-body bone mineral density values of people with celiac disease were significantly lower than those of people without it. After a year and a half on a gluten-free diet, the people with celiac disease were retested and it was found that their bone density had improved to the point where it was almost indistinguishable from that of the non-celiacs.[2]

Undetected celiac disease is associated with a forty- to hundredfold increased risk of intestinal lymphomas[3]—cancers of the lymphatic system. This is because in a person with celiac disease, the intestinal wall is constantly being irritated by gluten and the immune system doesn't fight cancer cells as well as it should. Over eighty international studies have been published on the increased incidence of cancer in people with this disease. In the case of intestinal lymphomas, once these have reached the point where they are diagnosed, the prognosis is generally very poor. But the good news is this: if celiac disease is diagnosed before these intestinal lymphomas become evident, and a gluten-free diet is strictly followed, the risk of developing this cancer decreases from a hundredfold back to near normal in just five years.

The prevention of cancer is the single most compelling argument for routine and repeated screening or monitoring for celiac disease in people with any of the above conditions, symptoms, or a close relative with the disease.

THE ONLY KNOWN CURE

The only known effective therapy for celiac disease is the complete, lifelong elimination of gluten from the diet. No wheat, rye, or barley in *any* form is allowed. Initially, we also recommend avoiding oats—but if an IgG food allergy test does not show the presence of oat antibodies, you could try reintroducing oats. Many health professionals allow oats to be eaten by their celiac patients. About 80 percent of celiac disease sufferers can tolerate oats.

If strictly followed, this regime swiftly and dramatically brings the sufferer back to health. Diseased intestines heal; deficient nutrients are again absorbed; bones get stronger; chronic pain disappears; body weight and muscle mass return to normal; the risk of intestinal cancer normalizes (see above); and even early thyroid disease disappears in some cases. But you have to suspect and diagnose celiac disease first!

Given that, it's wonderful that there has been a revolution in laboratory testing and screening for celiac disease. Hopefully, if these new tests are used intelligently, often—and soon—by health professionals, better health for the tens of millions of gluten-sensitive people around the world will be swiftly on its way.

Notes

Introduction

1. Royal College of Physicians special report, *Containing the Allergy Epidemic* (June 2003).

2. *U.S. News and World Report*, vol. 106, pp. 77 (1989).

3. Dixon, H., Treatment of delayed food allergy based on specific immunoglobulin G RAST testing, *Otolaryngol Head Neck Surgery*, vol. 1213, pp. 48–54; and independent scientific audit of 2,567 patients with long-term illnesses by the Department of Health Studies at the University of York, U.K., on behalf of the British Allergy Foundation. Study and fact sheet published 22 January 2001.

Chapter 1

1. Zuberbier, T. *et al.*, Department of Dermatology, Virchow-Klinikum, Humboldt University, Berlin, Germany, Pseudoallergen-free [food additive free] diet in the treatment of chronic urticaria, *Acta Derm Ventereol*, vol. 75, pp. 484–487 (1995).

Chapter 3

1. McDonald, P.J. *et al.*, Food protein-induced enterocolitis: Altered antibody response to ingested antigen, *Pediatr Res*, vol. 18, pp. 751–5 (1984).

2. Lindberg, E. *et al.*, Antibody (IgG, IgA, and IgM) to baker's yeast (*Saccharomyces cerevisiae*), yeast mannan, gliadin, ovalbumin and betalactoglobulin in monozygotic twins with inflammatory bowel disease, *Gut*, vol. 33, pp. 909–13 (1992).

3. Snook, J. and Shepherd, H. A., Bran supplementation in the treatment of irritable bowel syndrome, *Aliment Pharmacol Ther*, vol. 8, pp. 511–514 (1994).

4. Francis, C. Y. and Whorwell, P. J., Bran and irritable bowel syndrome: Time for reappraisal, *Lancet*, vol. 344, pp. 39–40 (1994).

5. Atkinson, W. *et al.*, Do food elimination diets improve Irritable Bowel Syndrome? A double blind trial based on IgG antibodies to food, *Gut*, vol. 53, pp. 1391–1393 (2004).

6. Sameer, Z. *et al.*, Food-specific serum IgG4 and IgE titers to common food antigens in irritable bowel syndrome, *Am J of Gastroenterol*, vol. 100, pp. 1550-1557 (2005).

7. Sameer, Z. *et al.*, Food-specific serum IgG4 and IgE titers to common food antigens in irritable bowel syndrome, *Am J of Gastroenterol*, vol. 100, pp. 1550-1557 (2005).

8. Wahnschaffe, U. *et al.*, Disease-like intestinal antibody pattern in patients with irritable bowel syndrome (IBS), *Gastroenterology*, vol. 114, pp. A430 (1998).

9. Wahnschaffe, U. *et al.*, Celiac disease-like abnormalities in a subgroup of patients with irritable bowel syndrome, *Gastroenterology*, vol. 121, pp. 1329-38 (2001).

10. Straus, S. E. *et al.*, Allergy and the chronic fatigue syndrome, *J Allergy Clin Immunol*, vol. 81 pp. 791-795 (1988).

11. Baraniuk, J. N. *et al.*, Rhinitis symptoms in chronic fatigue syndrome, *Ann Allergy Asthma Immunol*, vol. 81, pp. 359-365 (1998).

12. van den Bergh, V. *et al.*, Trigger factors in migraine, *Headache*, vol. 27, pp. 191-195 (1987).

13. Egger, J. *et al.*, Is migraine food allergy? A double-blind placebo-controlled trial of oligoantigenic diet treatment, *Lancet*, vol. 2, pp. 865-869 (1983).

14. Hughes, E. *et al.*, Migraine: A diagnostic test for etiology of food sensitivity by a nutritionally supported fast and confirmed by long term report, *Ann Allergy*, vol. 55, pp. 28-33 (1985).

15. Mansfield, L. *et al.*, Food allergy and adult migraine: Double-blind and mediator conformation of an allergic etiology, *Ann Allergy*, vol. 55, pp. 126-129 (1985).

16. van der Laar, M. A. and van der Korst, J. K., Food intolerance in rheumatoid arthritis I: A double blind, controlled trial of the clinical effects of elimination of milk allergens and azo dyes, *Ann Rheum Dis*, vol. 51, pp. 298-302 (1992); van der Laar, M. A. and van der Korst, J. K., Food intolerance in rheumatoid arthritis II: Clinical and histological aspects, *Ann Rheum Dis*, vol. 51, pp. 303-306 (1992).

17. Firer, M. A. *et al.*, Cow's milk allergy and eczema: Patterns of the antibody response to cow's milk in allergic skin disease, *Clin Allergy*, vol. 12, pp. 385-90 (1982).

18. Shakib, F. *et al.*, Relevance of milk- and egg-specific IgG4 in atopic eczema, *Int Arch Allergy Appl Immunol*, vol. 75, pp. 107-12 (1984); Shakib, F. *et al.*, Study of IgG sub-class antibodies in patients with milk intolerance, *Clin Allergy*, vol. 16, pp. 451-8 (1986).

19. Husby, S. *et al.*, IgG subclass antibodies to dietary antigens in atopic dermatitis, *Acta Derm Venereol Suppl*, vol. 144, pp. 88-92 (1989).

20. Iikura, Y. *et al.*, How to prevent allergic disease I. Study of specific IgE, IgG, and IgG4 antibodies in serum of pregnant mothers, cord blood, and infants, *Int Arch Allergy Appl Immunol*, vol. 88, pp. 250-2 (1989).

21. Lucarelli, S. *et al.*, Specific IgG and IgA antibodies and related subclasses in the

diagnosis of gastrointestinal disorders or atopic dermatitis due to cow's milk and egg, *Int J Immunopathol Pharmacol,* vol. 11, pp. 77–85 (1998).

22. Niggemann, B. *et al.,* Outcome of double-blind, placebo-controlled food challenge tests in 107 children with atopic dermatitis, *Clin Exp Allergy,* vol. 29, pp. 91–96 (1999).

23. Boushey, H. *et al.,* Daily versus as-needed corticosteroids for mild persistent asthma, *N Engl J Med.* 14 April, 352, pp. 1589–91 (2005).

24. Sicherer, S. H., and Leurg, D. Y., Advances in allergic skin disease, anaphylaxis, and hypersensitivity reactions to food, drugs, and insects, *J Allergy Clin Immunol,* vol. 116, pp. 153–63 (2005). Kanny, G., Atopic dermatitis in children and food allergy: combination or causality?, *Ann Dematol Venereol,* 132 Spec No. 1, 1590–103 (2005).

25. Danesch, U. C., Petasites hybridus (butterbur root) extract in the treatment of asthma—an open trial, *Altern Med Rev,* vol. 9, pp. 54–62 (2004).

26. Randolph, T., Allergy as a causative factor of fatigue, irritability and behaviour problems of children, *J Pediatr,* vol. 31, pp. 560 (1947).

27. Rowe, A., Allergic toxemia and fatigue, *Ann Allergy,* vol. 17, pp. 9 (1959).

28. Speer, F., ed., *Allergy of the Nervous System* (Thomas, 1970).

29. Campbell, M., Neurologic manifestations of allergic disease, *Ann Allergy,* vol. 31, pp. 485 (1973).

30. Hall, K., Allergy of the nervous system: A review, *Ann Allergy,* vol. 36, pp. 49–64 (1976).

31. Pippere, V., Some varieties of food intolerance in psychiatric patients, *Nutr Health,* vol. 3, pp. 125–136 (1984).

32. Pfeiffer, C. and Holford, P., *Mental Illness and Schizophrenia: The Nutrition Connection* (Thorsons, 1989).

33. Tuormaa, T., *An Alternative to Psychiatry* (The Book Guild, 1991).

34. Vlissides, D. *et al.,* A double-blind gluten-free/gluten-load controlled trial in a secure world population, *British Journal of Psychiatry,* vol. 148, pp. 447–52 (1986).

35. Jyonouchi, H. *et al.,* Dysregulated innate immune responses in young children with autism spectrum disorders: Their relationship to gastro-intestinal symptoms and dietary intervention, *Neuropsychobiology,* vol. 51, pp. 77–85 (2005).

36. Egger, J. *et al.,* Controlled trial of oligoantigenic diet treatment in the hyperkinetic syndrome, *Lancet,* vol. 1, pp. 540–545 (1985).

37. Feingold, B., Dietary management of behaviour and learning disabilities, in *Nutrition and Behavior,* S. A. Miller, ed. (Franklin Institute Press, 1981), p. 37.

Chapter 4

1. Egger, J. *et al.* (1985).

2. Carter, C. M. *et al.*, Effects of a few food diet in attention deficit disorder, *Arch Dis Child*, vol. 69, pp. 564–8 (1993).

3. Whiteley, P., Sunderland University Autism Unit, presentation to "Autism Unravelled" conference, London, May 2001.

4. Rosenfeld, R. M., What to expect from medical treatment of otitis media, *Pediatr Infect Dis J*, vol. 14, pp. 731–738 (1995).

5. Van den Broek, P. *et al.*, Letter to the editor, *Lancet*, vol. 348, p. 1517 (1996).

6. Williams, R. L. *et al.*, Use of antibiotics in preventing recurrent acute otitis media and in treating otitis media with effusion, *JAMA*, vol. 270, pp. 1344–1351 (1993).

7. Soutar, A., Bronchial reactivity and dietary antioxidants, *Thorax*, vol. 52, pp. 166–170 (1997).

8. Rebuffat, E. *et al.*, Difficulty in initiating and maintaining sleep associated with cow's milk allergy in infants, *Sleep*, vol. 10, pp. 116–121 (1987).

9. Kahn, A. *et al.*, Milk intolerance in children with persistent sleeplessness: A prospective double-blind crossover evaluation, *Pediatrics*, vol. 84, pp. 595–603 (1989).

10. Robson, W. L. *et al.*, Enuresis in children with attention-deficit hyperactivity disorder, *SC South Med J*, vol. 90, pp. 503–5 (1997).

11. Egger, J. *et al.*, Effect of diet treatment on enuresis in children with migraine or hyperkinetic behavior, *Clin Pediatr (Phila)*, vol. 31, pp. 302–307 (1992).

12. Scott, F. W. *et al.*, Potential mechanisms by which certain foods promote or inhibit the development of spontaneous diabetes in BB rats: Dose, timing, early effect on islet area, and switch in infiltrate from Th1 to Th2 cells, *Diabetes*, vol. 46, pp. 589–598 (1997).

13. Lorini, R. *et al.*, Clinical aspects of coeliac disease in children with insulin-dependent diabetes mellitus, *J Pediatr Endocrinol Metab*, Suppl 1, pp. 101–111 (1996).

14. Sjöberg, K. *et al.*, Screening for coeliac disease in adult insulin-dependent diabetes mellitus, *J Intern Med*, vol. 243, pp. 133–40 (1998).

15. Holmes, G. K. *et al.*, Coeliac disease and type 1 diabetes mellitus: The case for screening, *Diabet Med*, vol. 18, pp. 69–77 (2001).

16. Mohn, A. *et al.*, Celiac disease in children and adolescents with type I diabetes: Importance of hypoglycemia, *Pediatr Gastroenterol Nutr*, vol. 32, pp. 37–40 (2001).

17. Not, T. *et al.*, Undiagnosed celiac disease and risk of autoimmune disorders in subjects with type I diabetes, *Diabetologia*, vol. 44, pp. 151–5 (2001).

18. Kumar, V. *et al.*, Celiac disease-associated autoimmune endocrinopathies, *Diagn Lab Immunol*, vol. 8, pp. 678–85 (2001).

19. Ventura, A. *et al.*, Gluten-dependent diabetes-related and thyroid-related autoantibodies in patients with celiac disease, *J Pediatr*, vol. 137, pp. 263–265 (2000).

20. Toscano, V. *et al.*, Importance of gluten in the induction of endocrine autoanti-bodies and organ dysfunction in adolescent celiac patients, *Am J Gastroenterol,* vol. 95, pp. 1742-1748 (2000).

21. Kitts, D. *et al.*, Adverse reactions to food constituents: Allergy, intolerance, and autoimmunity, *Can J Physiol Pharmacol,* vol. 75, pp. 241-54 (1997).

Chapter 6

1. Cohen, G.A. *et al.*, Severe anemia and chronic bronchitis associated with a marked-ly elevated specific IgG to cow's milk protein, *Ann Allergy,* vol. 55, pp. 38-40 (1985).

2. Fallstrom, S. P. *et al.*, Serum antibodies against native, processed and digested cow's milk proteins in children with cow's milk protein intolerance, *Clin Allergy,* vol. 16, pp. 417-23 (1986).

3. Shakib, F. *et al.*, Study of IgG sub-class antibodies in patients with milk intolerance, *Clin Allergy,* vol. 16, pp. 451-8 (1986).

4. Host, A. *et al.*, Prospective estimation of IgG, IgG subclass and IgE antibodies to dietary proteins in infants with cow's milk allergy. Levels of antibodies to whole milk protein, BLG and ovalbumin in relation to repeated milk challenge and clinical course of cow's milk allergy, *Allergy,* vol. 47, pp. 218-29 (1992).

5. Hamburger, R. N. *et al.*, Long-term studies in prevention of food allergy: Patterns of IgG anti-cow's milk antibody responses, *Ann Allergy,* vol. 59, pp. 175-8 (1987).

6. Taylor, C. J. *et al.*, Detection of cow's milk protein intolerance by an enzyme-linked immunosorbent assay, *Acta Paediatr Scand,* vol. 77, pp. 49-54 (1988).

7. Iacono, G. *et al.*, IgG anti-beta lactoglubolin (beta lactotest): its usefulness in the diagnosis of cow's milk allergy, *It J Gastroentol,* vol. 27, pp. 355-360 (1995).

8. Cavataio, F. *et al.*, Gastroesophageal reflux associated with cow's milk allergy in infants: Which diagnostic examinations are useful?, *Am J Gastroenterol,* vol. 91, pp. 1215-20 (1996).

9. Duchateau, J. *et al.*, Anti-betalactoglobulin IgG antibodies bind to a specific profile of epitopes when patients are allergic to cow's milk proteins, *Clin Exp Allergy,* vol. 28, pp. 824-33 (1998).

10. U.S. National Institutes of Health (http://digestive.niddk.nih.gov/ddiseases/pubs/lactoseintolerance/)

11. Feskanich, D. *et al.*, Milk, dietary calcium, and bone fractures in women: A 12-year prospective study, *Am J Public Health,* vol. 87, pp. 992 (1997).

12. Paspati, I. *et al.*, Hip fracture epidemiology in Greece during 1977-1992, *Calcif Tissue Int,* vol. 62, pp. 542-547 (1998).

13. Lau, E. M. and Cooper, C., Epidemiology and prevention of osteoporosis in urban-ized Asian populations, *Osteoporosis,* vol. 3, pp. 23-26 (1993).

14. Fujita, T. and Fukase, M., Comparison of osteoporosis and calcium intake between Japan and the United States, *Proc Soc Exp Biol Med,* vol. 200, pp. 149-152 (1992).

15. Xu, L. *et al.,* Very low rates of hip fracture in Beijing, People's Republic of China: The Beijing Osteoprosis Project, *Am J Epedemiol,* vol. 144, pp. 901-907 (1996).

16. Torgerson, J. *et al.,* Randomised controlled trial of calcium and supplementation with cholecalciferol (vitamin D₃) for prevention of fractures in primary care, *BMJ,* vol. 330, pp. 1003 (2005).

17. Gerarduzzi, T. *et al.,* Celiac disease in USA among risk groups and general population in USA, *J Pediatr Gastroenterol Nutr,* vol. 31, pp. 104 (2000).

18. Sandiford, C. P. *et al.,* Identification of the major water/salt insoluble wheat proteins involved in cereal hypersensitivity, *Clin Exp Allergy,* vol. 27, pp. 1120-1129 (1997).

19. Högberg, L. *et al.,* Oats to children with newly diagnosed coeliac disease: A randomised double blind study, *Gut,* vol. 53, pp. 649-654 (2004).

20. Størsrud, S. *et al.,* Adult coeliac patients do tolerate large amounts of oats, *Eur J Clin Nutr,* vol. 57, pp. 163-169 (2003).

21. Cooke, S. K. and Sampson, H. A., Allergenic properties of ovomucoid in man, *J Immunol,* vol. 159, pp. 2026-2032 (1997).

22. Lever, R. *et al.,* Randomised controlled trial of advice on an egg exclusion diet in young children with atopic eczema and sensitivity to eggs, *Pediatr Allergy Immunol,* vol. 9, pp. 13-9 (1998).

23. Rance, F. and Dutau, G., Labial food challenge in children with food allergy, *Pediatr Allergy Immunol,* vol. 8, pp. 41-44 (1997).

24. Urisu, A. *et al.,* Allergenic activity of heated and ovomucoid-depleted egg white, *J Allergy Clin Immunol,* vol. 100, pp. 171-176 (1997).

25. Saxena, I. and Tayyab, S., Protein proteinase inhibitors from avian egg whites, *Cell Mol Life Sci,* vol. 53, pp. 13-23 (1997).

26. Atkinson, W. *et al.,* Food elimination based on IgG antibodies in irritable bowel syndrome: A randomised controlled trial, *Gut,* vol. 53, pp. 1459-64 (2004).

Chapter 7

1. Sblattero, D. *et al.,* Human recombinant tissue transglutaminase ELISA: An innovative diagnostic assay for celiac disease, *Am J Gastroenterol,* vol. 95, pp. 1253-1257 (2000).

Chapter 8

1. Jalonen, T., Identical permeability changes in children with different clinical manifestations of cow's milk allergy, *J Allergy Clin Immunol,* vol. 88, pp. 737-742 (1991).

2. Wagner, R. D. *et al.*, Biotherapeutic effects of probiotic bacteria on candidiasis in immunodeficient mice, *Infect Immun*, vol. 65, pp. 4165-4172 (1997).

3. Matsuzaki, T. and Chin, J., Modulating immune responses with probiotic bacteria, *Immunol Cell Biol*, vol. 78, pp. 67-73 (2000).

4. Majamaa, H. and Isolauri, E., Probiotics: A novel approach in the management of food allergy, *J Allergy Clin Immunol*, vol. 99, pp. 179-185 (1997).

5. Zheng, T. *et al.*, Lactation reduces breast cancer risk in Shandong Province, China, *Am J Epidemiol*, vol. 152, pp. 1129-1135 (2000).

6. Tomkins, A., Malnutrition, morbidity and mortality in children and their mothers, *Proc Nutr Soc*, vol. 59, pp. 135-146 (2000).

7. Hoppu, U. *et al.*, Maternal diet rich in saturated fat during breastfeeding is associated with atopic sensitization of the infant, *Eur J Clin Nutr*, vol. 54, pp. 702-705 (2000).

8. Dandrifosse, G. *et al.*, Are milk polyamines preventive agents against food allergy? *Proc Nutr Soc*, vol. 59, pp. 81-6 (2000).

9. Jensen-Jarolim, E., research presented at World Allergy Organization's (WAO) Congress in Vancouver, Canada, 6-12 September 2003.

10. Johnson, C. *et al.*, Antibiotic exposure in early infancy and risk for childhood atopy, *J Allergy Clin Immunol*, vol. 115, pp. 1218-1224 (2005).

11. Tariq, S. M. *et al.*, The prevalence of and risk factors for atopy in early childhood: A whole population birth cohort study, *J Allergy Clin Immunol*, vol. 101, pp. 587-593 (1998).

12. Tariq, S. M. *et al.* (1998).

13. Vally, H. *et al.*, Alcoholic drinks: Important triggers for asthma, *J Allergy Clin Immunol*, vol. 105, pp. 462-7 (2000).

14. Butland, B. K. *et al.*, Diet, lung function, and lung function decline in a cohort of 2512 middle aged men, *Thorax*, vol. 55, pp. 102-108 (2000).

15. Forastiere, F. *et al.*, Consumption of fresh fruit rich in vitamin C and wheezing symptoms in children, *Thorax*, vol. 55, pp. 283-288 (2000).

16. Iack, P. *et al.*, *J Allergy Clin Immunol*, vol. 103, pp. 351-352 (1999).

17. Hodge, L. *et al.*, Consumption of oily fish and childhood asthma, *Med J Aust*, vol. 164, pp. 137-140 (1996).

18. Kankaanpää, P. *et al.*, Dietary fatty acids and allergy, *Ann Med*, vol. 31, pp. 282-287 (1999).

19. Soutar, A., Bronchial reactivity and dietary antioxidants, *Thorax*, vol. 52, pp. 166-170 (1997).

20. Mauskop, A. *et al.*, Intravenous magnesium sulfate relieves migraine attacks in patents with low serum ionized magnesium levels: A pilot study, *Clin Sci,* vol. 89, pp. 633-636 (1995).

21. Trauninger, A. *et al.*, Oral magnesium load test in patients with migraine, *Headache,* vol. 42, pp. 114-9 (2002).

22. Sprietsma, J. E., Modern diets and diseases: NO-zinc balance. Under Th1, zinc and nitrogen monoxide (NO) collectively protect against viruses, AIDS, autoimmunity, diabetes, allergies, asthma, infectious diseases, atherosclerosis and cancer, *Med Hypotheses,* vol. 53, pp. 6-16 (1999).

Appendix 4

1. Meloni, G. *et al.*, Subclinical coeliac disease in school children from northern Sardinia, *The Lancet,* vol. 353, p. 37 (1999).

2. Mora, S. *et al.*, Reversal of low bone density with a gluten-free diet in children and adolescents with celiac disease, *Am J Clin Nutr,* vol. 67, pp. 477-481 (1998).

3. Hoggan, R., Considering wheat, rye, and barley proteins as aids to carcinogens, *Med Hypotheses,* vol. 49, pp. 285-288 (1997).

Further Reading

Braly, James, and Ron Hoggan. *Dangerous Grains.* New York, NY: Avery, 2002.

Braly, James. *Food Allergy and Nutrition Revolution.* New Canaan, CT: Keats, 1992.

Braly, James, and Patrick Holford. *The H-Factor Solution.* North Bergen, NJ: Basic Health Publications, 2003.

Holford, Patrick. *New Optimum Nutrition Bible.* Berkeley, CA: Crossing Press, 2005.

Holford, Patrick. *Optimum Nutrition for the Mind.* North Bergen, NJ: Basic Health Publications, 2004.

Miller, Merlene, and David Miller. *Staying Clean and Sober.* Orem, UT: Woodland Publishing, 2005.

Resources

The American Academy of Environmental Medicine (AAEM)

AAEM is an international association of physicians and other professionals interested in the clinical aspects of man and his environment. The founders and members of AAEM are recognized as the first to describe or the first organization to acknowledge food allergy/food addiction, rotary diversified diet, chemically less-contaminated foods, yeast syndrome, and chronic fatigue and fibromyalgia syndromes.

Contact information:
AAEM
7701 E Kellogg Dr., Suite 625
Wichita, KS 67207-1705
Phone: (316) 684-5500
Website: www.aaem.com

The American College for Advancement in Medicine (ACAM)

ACAM is a not-for-profit medical society dedicated to educating physicians and other healthcare professionals on the latest findings and emerging procedures in preventive/nutritional medicine. ACAM's goals are to improve skills, knowledge, and diagnostic procedures as they relate to complementary and alternative medicine; to support research; and to develop awareness of alternative methods of medical treatment. To find an ACAM physician well schooled in nutrition and allergy, visit the ACAM website or call the number listed below. Dr. Braly is an active member of ACAM.

Contact information:
ACAM
23121 Verdugo Drive, Suite 204
Laguna Hills, CA 92653
Phone: 1-888-439-6891
Website: www.acam.org/dr_search

Other nutrition- and food-allergy-oriented organizations include:

International and American Associations of Clinical Nutritionists (IAACN)
16775 Addison Road, Suite 100
Addison, TX 75001
Phone: 972-407-9089
Website: www.iaacn.org

Society for Orthomolecular Health Medicine (OHM)
2698 Pacific Avenue
San Francisco, CA 94115
Phone: 415-922-6462
Fax: 415-346-2519
E-mail: sohma@aol.com

International Society for Orthomolecular Medicine (ISOM)
16 Florence Ave.
Toronto, Ontario
Canada M2N 1E9
Phone: 416-733-2117
Website: www.orthomed.org

NEWSLETTER

Holford Wellness Advisor Newsletter
Subscribe to Patrick Holford's *Wellness Advisor* newsletter for monthly guidance on achieving super health, including review and analysis of the latest research. A one-year subscription (12 issues) is $39.95. Call 800-809-9610 or order online at www.holfordhealth.com. Sign up for Patrick Holford's free health e-letter at www.holfordhealth.com.

LABORATORY TESTS

Food Allergy Tests: York, England–based YorkTest Laboratories
YorkTest Laboratories has been established for more than twenty years and is one of the world's leading quality providers of IgG food-allergy testing and screening for celiac disease. YorkTest provides you with an easy and convenient service in which you can take your blood sample in the comfort of your own home by means of a simple pinprick. In the YorkTest's package provided to you, your blood sample can then safely be sent back to YorkTest Laboratories in York, England, for a full food-allergy test. YorkTest provides the *food-*

SCAN Food Intolerance 113 Food Test or the *foodSCAN Food Intolerance 42 Food Intolerance Test.* You will also receive a comprehensive guidebook with either test, which will help to explain the results and offer recommendations. The results of your test are also presented in a handy credit card-sized format you can carry with you. Visit their website (see below) for more information and how to order their test packages.

> *Contact information:*
> YORKTEST Laboratories Ltd.
> York Science Park
> York
> YO10 5DQ
> United Kingdom
> Phone: 011 44 1904 428579*
> Fax: 011 44 1904 422000*
> E-mail: ynl@allergy-testing.com
> Website: www.yorktest.com or www.allergy-testing.com
> *When calling from the United States, remember to compensate for the different time zone.*

Food Allergy Tests: Immuno Laboratories, Inc. (in partnership with Better Health USA)

Immuno Laboratories, Inc., provides reproducible, reliable food allergy testing either through your personal physician or through the Immuno Labs physician referral service. And, they offer support from a team of nutritionists familiar with food allergy testing and rotation diets. They offer a guarantee that if you don't feel noticeably better after ninety days on their program, they will refund your testing fee.

> *Contact information:*
> Immuno Laboratories, Inc.
> 6801 Powerline Road
> Fort Lauderdale, FL 33309
> Phone: 954-691-2500 or 800-231-9197
> Fax: 954-691-2505

Gluten Sensitivity and Celiac Disease Tests: Prometheus Laboratories, Inc.

State-of-the-art testing for gluten sensitivity and celiac disease is offered by Prometheus Laboratories, Inc. No laboratory today is offering a more comprehensive evaluation.

Contact information:
Prometheus Laboratories, Inc.
9410 Carroll Park Drive
San Diego, CA 92121
Phone: 858-824-0895 or 888-423-5227
Fax: 858-824-0896
Website: www.prometheus-labs.com

Intestinal Permeability Assessment: Great Smokies Diagnostic Laboratory
The Intestinal Permeability Assessment by Great Smokies directly measures the ability of two nonmetabolized sugar molecules—mannitol and lactulose—to permeate the intestinal mucous membrane. Mannitol is easily absorbed and serves as a marker of transcellular uptake, while lactulose is only slightly absorbed and serves as a marker for mucosal leakiness. To perform the test, you are asked to mix premeasured amounts of lactulose and mannitol and drink the mixture. The test by Great Smokies then measures the amount of lactulose and mannitol recovered in a urine sample.

Contact information:
Great Smokies Laboratories
63 Zillico Street
Asheville, NC 28801
Phone: 828-253-0621 or 800-522-4762.
Fax: (828) 252-9303
Website: www.gsdl.com

ADDICTION TREATMENT CENTERS WITH EMPHASIS ON NUTRITIONAL INTERVENTION

Bridging the Gaps, Inc.
Bridging the Gaps, Inc., provides traditional psychosocial treatment as well as science-based alternatives, including dietary counseling, oral supplementation, and intravenous-oral nutrient therapy for people seeking successful recovery from alcohol, drug addictions, and related mental health issues. Their focus includes physiological and biochemical rebalancing for the individual by exploring the nutritional and environmental aspects of treatment, in addition to the emotional, spiritual, and social factors involved—a truly integrative approach to a multifactor disease.

Contact information:
Bridging the Gaps, Inc.
423 West Cork Street
Winchester, VA 22601
Phone: 540-535-1111 or 866-711-1234
Fax: 540-450-1205
Website: www.bridgingthegaps.com

Health Recovery Center (HRC)

HRC has pioneered an approach to treatment of addiction based on achieving biochemical balance, without prescription drugs. In conjunction with physicians, HRC assesses and restores physical health via medical appointments, laboratory tests, and nutritional counseling.

Contact information:
Health Recovery Center
3255 Hennepin Ave. South
Minneapolis, MN 55408
Phone: 612-827-7800 or 800-554-9155
E-mail: businessoffice@healthrecovery.com
Website: www.healthrecovery.com

Miller Associates

David and Merlene Miller are a husband-and-wife team with over twenty-five years of experience in the field of addictions, ADHD, and relapse prevention. They have worked not only as counselors and consultants, but also in the academic field as associate professors who teach and develop curricula for addiction study programs leading to a bachelor's degree. They are among the leading pioneers, authors, and spokespeople in the area of nutrition and addictions (see their most recent book, the award-winning *Staying Clean and Sober,* Woodland Publishing, 2005). They provide a national referral service to health consumers and professionals looking to further their education in the field of addiction or who may be searching for addiction treatment centers offering food allergy management, dietary counseling, and intravenous and oral nutrient therapy in the treatment of alcohol, drug, and food addiction, and prevention of relapse.

Contact information:
Miller Associates
Phone: 800-287-0906
Website: www.Miller-Associates.org

Index

About the Authors

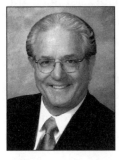 **James Braly, M.D.**, graduated from St. Louis University School of Medicine in 1970 and has remained at the cutting edge of new American medical research in natural medicine and laboratory science for the past twenty-four years.

Disenchanted with prescription drugs and symptom-oriented treatments, Dr. Braly founded innovative naturopathic medical clinics in Encino and San Mateo, California (1980–1994), specializing in an optimum-nutrition approach to healthcare, backed up by proper laboratory testing. He founded and directed one of the first federally licensed clinical laboratories in the world for testing delayed-onset IgG-based food intolerance. Both through his clinics and laboratory, Dr. Braly supervised the treatment of thousands of people using nutrition-based, nondrug treatments for preventing and reversing disease.

He was one of the first doctors to alert us to the epidemic of IgG-mediated food allergies and is the author of the best-selling book *Dr. Braly's Food Allergy and Nutrition Revolution.* He is also a recognized world authority of celiac disease and has helped to research and expose the widespread problem of gluten sensitivity, culminating in his recent book, *Dangerous Grains.* He is medical editor and consultant for www.drbralyallergyrelief.com, a website specializing in consumer education about clinical nutrition, delayed-onset food allergy, gluten sensitivity, and celiac disease. He is currently involved as medical director, researcher, lecturer, and product formulator with Laguna Hills, California–based LifeStream Recovery, Inc., a company that specializes in the research, development, and implementation of integrative psychosocial, dietary, nutritional, and herbal-based treatments for addictions and neurodegenerative diseases.

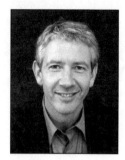

Patrick Holford is a leading light in new approaches to health and nutrition. He started his academic career in the field of psychology. While completing his bachelor's degree in experimental psychology at the University of York, he researched the role of nutrition in mental health and illness and later tested the effects of improved nutrition on children's IQ—an experiment that was the subject of a Horizon documentary in 1987. He became a student of two-time Nobel Prize winner Dr. Linus Pauling, who believed that the future of medicine was "optimum nutrition."

In 1984, with the support of Dr. Pauling, Patrick Holford founded the Institute for Optimum Nutrition (ION). A charitable and independent educational trust for furthering education and research in nutrition, ION is now one of the most respected training colleges for clinical nutritionists. At ION he pioneered many radical ideas in nutrition, from the importance of antioxidants to the dangers of HRT.

He has written more than twenty popular books, now translated into seventeen languages. The first, *The Optimum Nutrition Bible,* has sold more than 1 million copies worldwide.

THE H-FACTOR SOLUTION

JAMES BRALY, M.D., & PATRICK HOLFORD

Homocysteine Is the Best Single Indicator of Whether You Are Likely to Live Long or Die Young.

How to Add 20 Years to Your Life and Life to Your Years with 12 Simple Lifestyle Changes

THE
H.*
FACTOR
SOLUTION

*(Homocysteine, the Best Single Indicator of Whether You Are Likely to Live Long or Die Young)

JAMES BRALY, M.D.
& PATRICK HOLFORD

Staying healthy, happy, clearheaded, and full of energy into old age—this is what we all want. But insuring that we do depends on how well we can "read" the state of our health. What if there was a single test that could do that, as well as point the way to a superhealthy future? Fortunately, there is. This test measures your level of homocysteine, an amino acid that is found naturally in the blood.

High levels of homocysteine, or a high "H score," predicts your risk of more than 100 diseases and medical conditions, including Alzheimer's disease, cardiovascular disease, cancer, and depression. In fact, it is even more accurate than a cholesterol reading for predicting the risk of a heart attack or stroke. It also is the single best functional indicator of folate, B_{12}, and B_6 vitamin status. When homocysteine is high, one or more of these vitamins is low. Moreover, elevated homocysteine is an excellent biological marker for glutathione, SAME, L-cysteine, and methyl donor deficiencies; when homocysteine is high, one or more of these critical anti-aging, health-promoting natural body chemicals is deficient.

In *The H-Factor Solution,* best-selling authors Dr. James Braly and Patrick Holford clearly explain what factors contribute to a high H score and how you can go about dramatically lowering your level to a risk-free range with simple dietary changes and nutrient supplementation. They also describe exciting advancements in laboratory testing and provide a clear definition of the optimal range for homocysteine.

Based on groundbreaking research, this informative book is your guide to a superhealthy H score. Knowing your score and taking the appropriate steps to lower it and keep it low can add quality years to your life.

U.S. $14.95 / Can. $23.95 • 256 pages • 6" x 9" paperback • ISBN: 1-59120-042-3 / 978-1-59120-042-0

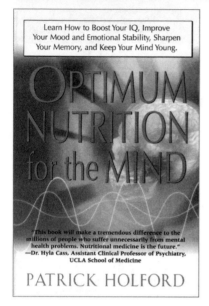

Learn How to Boost Your IQ, Improve Your Mood and Emotional Stability, Sharpen Your Memory, and Keep Your Mind Young.

"This book will make a tremendous difference to the millions of people who suffer unnecessarily from mental health problems. Nutritional medicine is the future."
—Dr. Hyla Cass, Assistant Clinical Professor of Psychiatry, UCLA School of Medicine

PATRICK HOLFORD

OPTIMUM NUTRITION for the MIND
PATRICK HOLFORD

"Optimum Nutrition for the Mind gives us a most powerful weapon in our fight against mental disease. It is also essential reading for anyone wanting to stay in top mental health throughout life, free from depression, memory decline, and, even worse, senility."
—Abram Hoffer, M.D., Ph.D.

How we think and feel is directly affected by what we take into our bodies. Although it may seem strange, eating the right food has been proven to boost IQ, improve mood and emotional stability, sharpen the memory, and keep the mind young. Similarly, the harmful things we take into our bodies, or anti-nutrients—including oxidants, alcohol, sugar, and stimulants—negatively impact mental health. These are the main issues world-renowned author Patrick Holford discusses in *Optimum Nutrition for the Mind.*

The book is broken down into eight parts. Part 1 provides "food for thought"—what are the best foods to eat and which nutrients are most bene-ficial. Part 2 discusses how to protect the brain from becoming polluted and how to identify and avoid "brain allergies." Part 3 teaches readers how to boost their intelligence, enhance their memories, beat the blues, solve sleep problems, and more. Part 4 turns to mental illness, Part 5 to depression and schizophrenia, and Parts 6 and 7 to mental health in the young and old, respectively. These parts include information on identifying and understanding specific problems and how to treat them naturally and effectively. Part 8 provides a complete action plan for regaining and maintaining good mental health. The book closes with a helpful Resources section that provides readers with useful addresses.

From boosting one's memories, solving depression, and beating addictions to overcoming eating disorders, preventing age-related memory decline, and balancing out mood swings, *Optimum Nutrition for the Mind* covers a wide range of important topics and will be of interest to anyone who wants to think and feel great.

U.S. $17.95 / Can. $28.95 • 400 pages • 6" x 9" paperback • ISBN: 1-59120-105-2 / 978-1-59120-105-2